— THE —
Sexual
MAN

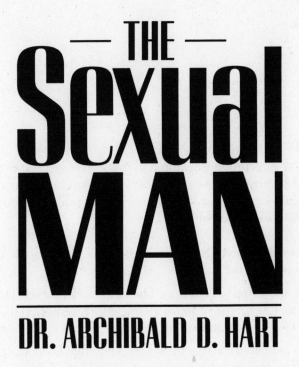

THE
Sexual
MAN

DR. ARCHIBALD D. HART

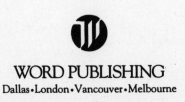

WORD PUBLISHING
Dallas•London•Vancouver•Melbourne

THE SEXUAL MAN

Library of Congress Cataloging-in-Publication Data

Hart, Archibald D.
    The sexual man : masculinity without guilt / Archibald D. Hart.
      p.   cm.
    ISBN 0-8499-1076-5 (hardcover); ISBN 0-8499-3684-5 (trade paper)
    1. Men—Sexual behavior.   2. Masculinity (Psychology)   3. Sex (Psychology)   4. Sex—Religious aspects—Christianity.   I. Title.
HQ28.H37
155.3'32—dc20   93–50132
                                                                          CIP

Printed in the United States of America

11 12 13 14 15 QPV 03 02 01 00 99

To Archibald Daniel Hart, my grandfather. I not only
inherited his name but also his personality
and temperament—for which I am
unabashedly thankful.

Contents

List of Figures

Acknowledgments

My profoundest appreciation goes to all those who have helped me bring this project to completion, especially to:

- Kip Jordon and Ernie Owen for entrusting me with this study.

- The many men, especially clergy, who responded to my call for subjects.

- Lavonne Schaasfma, my graduate student, who helped me with the difficult task of entering data into that miracle of modern times, the computer.

- Nova Hutchins, my executive secretary, for hours upon hours of meticulous and loving care given to the shaping of this manuscript.

- Lela Gilbert for her patience in editing the manuscript.

- To my daughters Sharon, Catherine, and Sylvia, as well as their husbands Richard, Rick, and Russ, for their help, honest feedback, and contributions to this book.

- To my wife, Kathleen, who has helped me achieve a lot of growth and movement toward my own sexual healthiness, even though I had such a bad start as a boy.

Introduction

My need to write this book emerged out of more than twenty-five years of work with men. These have been men whom I consider to be relatively "normal." Yet, for one reason or another, they struggle to understand their sexuality.

No matter what the context of my encounter, these men seemed confused. They tended either to shut up or to guiltily beg for pardon whenever they were confronted with the subject of sex. Whether I met them after a lecture, in a seminar, in my therapy office, or simply in private conversation, the issues, conflicts, and questions seemed always to be the same. They had difficulty distinguishing what is normal and healthy from what is sick and dysfunctional. They struggled to differentiate between ordinary and common feelings about sex and what is bizarre or deviant. Many feared that their strong sexual drive was in some way a distortion of nature. They even feared that they had developed a perverted sexuality. Many reported that their wives had made statements like, "You're a sex addict; no normal man could want sex as much as you do," or "Go see a doctor. There's something wrong with your sexual obsession."

Feeling as if they are struggling to keep their heads above turbulent waves of testosterone, most men report a tremendous conflict to control their sex drive. They feel driven by their hormones and find that their God-given sexuality, rather than being a delight and source of vitality, has been forced into a dark secret filled with shame, frustration, and anger. Their struggle keeps them unhappy, robs them of complete fulfillment in life, and very frequently destroys their marriages.

A major factor in many marital breakups is a failure to work out a mutually satisfying sexual relationship. A mismatch between husbands' and wives' sexual needs, unless worked out in a way that satisfies both, spells doom to marital happiness. The emotional and biological forces at work in sexuality are powerful and cannot be minimized.

I have chosen to focus my attention on a special group of our male population. I call them "good men." They are the men who make up the middle of the road. They are mainstream men. Mostly they are married, fathers, church-going, God-fearing, decent, hard-working, honest men doing ordinary living.

Why study and write about such men? Because they make up the vast majority of the males in our world. They are not kinky or weird in their sexuality. They are good men with good families, good kids, and good values. They care about being good. They try to live balanced lives, are considerate of others, and desire to be healthy in all areas of their being. And by and large they succeed, except in their struggle with sexuality. Yet they are very conscious of their sexuality because they want to be good. Other men don't care to try; these men do. So I have chosen to discuss the sexuality of these ordinary men.

There is another important reason why I want to write about these men. Every time I hear or read about the latest study or report on what is happening to male sexuality in our time, I am struck by how irrelevant much of the report is to me as a man. These studies, as I will show later in this book, tend to be preoccupied with the fringe issues of sexuality. Their preoccupation seems to be with how we are pushing back the boundaries of normality as far as it will go. They focus on questions like: How many men dabble in cross-dressing? Who indulges in sadomasochism? Who cheats on his wife? And, of course, there is always the question of how the AIDS epidemic is impacting the bedroom.

Now, I'm not saying that some or all of these issues aren't important. They are. But they leave me, along with millions of other men, stone cold. I am not interested, personally, in how many sexual partners the average male has had by the age of twenty-five, or whether men have sex at work. Most studies of sexuality only want to know about deviancy and sexual disorders. They're really not all that interested in what it means to be normal. I am more interested in how ordinary men struggle with their sexuality, because that is where I am: monogamous, mainstream, and modest—and not ashamed of it.

This book, then, has its limits. It does not address in any depth the sexual perversions or deviations except to clarify what is considered to be normal. It is not a broad-based study of male sexuality, but a very focused report on heterosexuality. The topic of homosexuality is very important, but it is too vast and complex to be treated cursorily; so I have chosen not to address it here. It would detract from my primary purpose, which is to help heterosexual men understand their sexual experiences in healthier ways.

The male sex drive is a force so powerful that it can easily be misdirected and misshapen. Most of the men I have studied come from a religious background, because I am interested in knowing how religion influences, for good or bad, our sexuality. And I hardly ever encounter a good man who doesn't have some sexual damage because of a deeply rooted, false sense of guilt. Many have learned to ignore it, but it is there nevertheless, working its damage in the background.

Finally, this is not a book about sexual morals, although I cannot deny that my own values as a Christian husband, father, and grandfather will show through. My intention, however, is not to judge or condemn, but to describe and try to define the boundaries of what it means to be normal. No doubt this will disappoint some readers who would want me to mount a tirade against sexual sin, but that is not my purpose. Most of the good men I know are already too hard on themselves as it is when it comes to sex. They feel guilty for being normal, and they rob themselves of much-needed self-esteem. I trust that what I have to share in this book will help a few of them understand themselves and come to terms with how God has made them. Perhaps that will enable them to rest content in the knowledge that they are, in fact, perfectly and completely normal.

Archibald D. Hart, Ph.D.

1

Male Sexuality—The Untold Story

Sex is joyous, yet perplexing. Transcendent, yet troublesome. Of all life's experiences, it is probably the most bewildering. While men think about sex dozens of times every living day, they don't like to discuss it. In fact, they usually don't talk about it, unless they're talking dirty.

Should we talk about sex? Absolutely. For one thing, when we don't talk about our sexuality, our silence breeds distortions. Things that are kept silent somehow seem corrupted, misguided, and even immoral. As we talk to each other we increase our understanding, and we keep the beauty of sex intact.

When it comes to male sex, let's stop pretending everything is all right. The truth is that most men in our culture are in serious trouble. Despite the sexual revolution, or perhaps because of it, men today are becoming more and more confused about this most primal aspect of their being. They don't have a clue about what it is to be normal, and they can't figure out why women don't understand their preoccupation with sex.

Our ideas about male sexuality have changed drastically over the past thirty years. This radical change has left many men with only a vague idea of their true role and identity as sexual beings in today's society. Sex has become an end in itself, not a means to an end. And for many men, sex is a dead-end street.

Superficially, there is much concerned talk. We hear how men can become sexually addicted. How sexual perversions take root in early years. How men are the main perpetrators of sexual abuse in the home and of sexual harassment in the workplace. Men are losing their sexual spontaneity and naturalness by being forced to be self-conscious and self-monitoring in ways that never previously existed.

A new sexual self-consciousness is taking root. It takes its toll in many ways, some we don't readily recognize. For instance, because of increased reports about child sexual abuse, fathers don't know how to relate to their daughters anymore. There was a time when you could just be yourself—romp, tease, and play games. We can't do that so easily these days. Too much close physical contact might be misinterpreted as sexual, so fathers pull back and become distant, even cold, leaving their daughters without a father's emotional warmth.

Meanwhile, grandfathers don't like being left alone with their grand-daughters for fear they might be suspected of sexual abuse. Countless grandfathers have even been accused of child molestation simply because some overzealous therapist has misinterpreted an obscure story, night-mare, dreams, or unaccountable anger as being related to an incident in a child's life. In most cases these accusations have proven false, yet the damage done by a mere accusation can never be repaired or removed. So grandfathers, uncles, cousins, and even family friends prefer to keep their distance from little girls.

Some men in the workplace have stopped being gentlemanly or say-ing nice things to their female colleagues. Men dare not compliment a new hairstyle or dress, no matter how innocently they do it, for fear that at some future time this compliment will come to haunt them as an ac-cusation of sexual harassment. Many managers who have tried to dismiss a female employee have reaped what they have sown in earlier years.

On the dating scene men are fearful about how to respond to close physical contact. I'm not talking about a lecherous man trying to seduce a date. I'm concerned about honorable men who genuinely want to build a relationship. They struggle to determine what is appropriate, fearing the possibility of arousal if they get too close. The only way they know how to control their sexual feelings is to pull back, remain distant, and become clumsy. Their testosterone fog turns them into jerks, not red-blooded, healthy males seeking to find and win a compatible life partner.

Men stereotypically have great difficulty getting in touch with their deeper feelings. They tend to run away from really trying to understand themselves. Now they are being forced to run and hide even more. And, tragically, they bear their confusion in silence. As the research I will report demonstrates, men talk to no one about their deep, sexual feelings, least of all to their own wives or friends.

I think it's time we took a look at the hidden side of male sexuality and explored the deep secrets of average males. I am sure God never intended sexuality to become as distorted and feared as it is today. Something has gone terribly wrong, and in order to fix it, we first must try to understand it.

Frank's Untold Story

There are some men who are perfectly comfortable and totally satisfied with their sexuality—not a lot, but some. A few genuinely feel they have discovered great fulfillment and deep satisfaction in their sexual life. I count myself fortunate to be in this group. For these men, satisfaction has nothing to do with quantity, but quality. It doesn't depend entirely on their partner, either. Their secret is simply this: they have resolved their own sexual hang-ups.

In my clinical work and the many seminars I have taught over the years, I have learned that this is not the way the vast majority of men feel. Frank's story is representative of many men.

A lawyer in his early thirties, Frank was raised in a deeply religious mid-western home. He never resented his family's faith; in fact, he had come to value it greatly. Frank never gave much thought to his sexuality until his marriage began to disintegrate. In his despair, he wrote me the following letter:

> For years I have punished myself for having sexual desires, especially if I felt those desires toward someone other than my wife. I was taught that when you are married you lose all sexual feelings toward other women. I now realize how stupid this is. I have never been unfaithful to my wife, whom I love dearly, but I just don't seem to be able to stop my sexual feelings from

running amuck. I don't want these feelings; they are driving
me crazy. But I don't seem to be able to get rid of them. The
harder I try the stronger they become. What is it with this
sexual stuff? The more you try to forget or ignore it the more it
drives you crazy.

Now don't jump to any conclusions or condemn Frank's struggles as
immature or atypical. And don't be quick to blame his parents for faulty
teaching or his religious upbringing for distorting his sexuality, either.
That might be true in some cases, but not in Frank's. Frank's parents, even
by his own account, were balanced, healthy, and nonjudgmental people,
and they tried to raise their children that way.

Frank grew up on a farm, and he had watched animals copulate before he
was old enough to spit. His parents talked openly about sexuality and laid no
guilt trips on him about masturbation, or anything else for that matter. From
everything I could determine Frank had a normal, healthy upbringing.

So where had things gone wrong?

After many months of careful exploration it appeared to me that
Frank's confusion about his sexuality arose from one primary source: He
had no idea how common and ordinary his feelings were. He always
thought he was the exception. Watching animals and hearing the facts of
sex provide information, but they don't help a boy, and later a man, understand the sexual storm that rages within. None of Frank's early instruction
addressed the deeper feelings and experiences of sexuality in the male.

Frank had come to believe that the strength of his sex drive was abnormal and that his mind's preoccupation with sexual ideas was inappropriate.
He could not reconcile his attractions to women with his desire to be a
good husband and a healthy father. Since no one talked about these matters, he thought he must be the odd one out!

"If people really knew what thoughts were going on in my head, they'd
have me sent to the nearest loony farm," he said to me once. Typically, the
more Frank struggled to overcome his sexual thoughts and feelings,
the more obsessional they became.

By never talking to other men, Frank missed the one real truth that
could have set him free from guilt and confusion: *Strong sexual feelings are
common to all normal men. They are determined more by hormones than by
evil desire. They are not sinful in and of themselves.*

Frank's misery was exacerbated by one further problem. He and his wife were miles apart in their sexual needs. She clearly suffered from what is now being called a hypoactive sexual desire disorder—she simply had no desire for sex.

This hadn't always been the case, but for several years Frank's wife had found sex unappealing, even revolting. To defend herself against Frank's approaches she started to label her husband as a "sex-crazed maniac." Obviously, this made Frank feel terrible about himself, so he stopped reaching out for sex. By the time I saw Frank, he hadn't had sex for months and months and the couple's marriage relationship was in serious trouble.

To her credit, Frank's wife was the first to seek help after noticing how angry her husband had become. She responded positively to feedback about Frank's condition. Together they were not only able to save their marriage, but also to reverse her low sexual desire, which involved the aftereffects of childbearing, stress, and depression. By the way, stress and depression can also be a common cause of low sexual desire in men, so this is not just a female problem.

The Nature of Male Sexuality

Like Frank, the average normal male thinks about sex more often than he cares to admit. Men often wake up thinking about it, and they go to bed thinking about it. Immediately after being sexually satisfied, the normal male may be able to focus elsewhere—for a while. But it is just a matter of time before his thoughts lead him back to sex. And I'm talking about the preacher as much as the truckdriver.

Sure, the average man thinks of other things, like football and politics, but eventually all mental roads lead back to this one central fixation: Sex. There are times when the obsession fades and even vanishes. Give him an intense challenge at work. Let him buy a new computer or sports car. Give him a golf bag or a fishing trip. He'll forget about sex for a while. But sooner or later, like a smoldering fire, it will flare up again. Strong, urgent, forceful, and impatient, the sex drive dominates the mind and body of every healthy male. Like it or not, that's the way it is.

And I'm talking about men in their sixties, seventies, or even eighties, as well as about teenagers. In fact, over the years I have talked with dozens of men in their eighties, and they have reminded me in no uncertain terms that their sexual feelings have not changed at all as they've aged. Frequency may subside, but not desire.

Deeply religious men may try to deny it, but they can be just as obsessed with sex as hard-core pornography addicts. I know. I counsel scores of pastors, missionaries, and other religious workers who are hung up on sex. They are just as human as everyone else.

Why doesn't religion remove these sexual feelings? Because religious men have the same physical bodies as everyone else, and the sex drive is primarily a matter of hormones. Getting religious may help with control, but it clearly doesn't take sexual desire away. Some of us probably wish our sexuality weren't so primitive and biological, but it is. There's no purpose to be served in trying to dress it up with idealism.

To make matters worse, our culture has come to glorify sex. And by defining what is and isn't good sex, the media has distorted it. Movies, TV, and magazines continue to feed this distortion. I would even go so far as to suggest that as a culture, our Western world has "neuroticized sexuality." We have turned good, otherwise healthy males into compulsive masturbators and obsessional addicts. If something isn't done to turn this around, I fear for the next century.

The Struggle for Control

From the moment the sex hormones start to flow, the male begins a battle. It is a battle for control, and the male who doesn't engage in this battle is dangerous to women and society. Many rapists, for instance, are men who have given up struggling to control their sex drive. Sadists and even sexual serial killers have done the same. But what about ordinary boys and men? For almost every male of every age, the sex drive is a powerful and urgent feeling, demanding his immediate attention.

Why is it important to define the boundaries of normal and to encourage a healthy approach to control the sexual drive? Very simply because most men, especially Christian men, feel that there is something wrong with them. And while the vast majority of these men never do anything disgraceful, their inner struggle is not without its pain and penalties. They feel guilty and shameful; their self-esteem is often eroded because they become obsessed with sexual fantasies or attractions. Lust becomes a war within, an ongoing battle that seems to have no possibility for victory. And they know all too well that those who have stopped fighting it have stopped being good men.

For the highly moral male with strong Christian or other religious leanings, the effort to control sexual impulses is particularly demoralizing. We long to be free of unnecessary temptation. We love the sexual feelings but hate the things these feelings want us to do. Hormones don't always respond to cold showers or watching football games. Even excessive exercise only provides partial relief. In fact, most health and exercise emporiums, so popular today, only serve to expose us to females in tight clothing. Their undulating bodies more than counteract the sublimating effects of a hard workout. Everywhere you turn, you just can't escape being exposed to erotic stimuli.

Females Who Don't Understand

Let me highlight one further aggravating problem that makes the development of adequate control in the male difficult. Many women don't understand the male sex drive. They are generally less obsessed with sex than men are and don't develop the same compulsiveness about it. Some women seem to have fewer struggles; still others don't seem to need sex at all. Strange, isn't it, how the sexes in general can be so different?

Some women, further, are naive about their appearance and behavior. They dress provocatively, perhaps to attract a particular male. They seem to expect other men, for whom the provocation is not intended, to turn a blind eye. These women don't seem to understand that all men are turned on by revealing dresses, short skirts, evocative perfume, or close proximity.

If women do not want to be treated as sex objects in the workplace, they should consider their habit of dressing seductively. Of course, men are ultimately responsible for their own sexuality, and there is never any excuse for harassment. However, a later section of this book will be devoted to helping women understand how men on the job think about sex, how and what excites them, and what women should do if they want to avoid sexual harassment.

In fact, I hope the pages that follow have as much appeal for women as for men. Just as men need to understand themselves, it would also be helpful for women to understand the male sex drive. Better understanding can only bring a richer relationship between the sexes.

My Research and Study

A brief description of my research for this book is necessary before I can proceed further. Other major research projects that have examined sexuality (Kinsey, Masters and Johnson, and Janus) have taken too broad a look at too wide a spectrum of sexual experiences. For the purposes of this book, I have chosen to examine a much narrower aspect. As I've said before, my focus, intentionally, is to examine the sexual experience of mainstream, middle-of-the-road, normal, heterosexual men.

There are four major sources for the data I will incorporate into this report on normal male sexuality: clinical psychotherapy interviews, confidential papers of clergy students, questionnaires, and other studies.

First, there is the data I have gleaned from more than twenty-five years of in-depth interviews as a psychotherapist with men, many of whom were clergy. This clinical base of knowledge is far more comprehensive than can be gathered from a larger sampling of males where only questionnaires are used.

Historically, clinical studies such as this have always been invaluable in providing information about a broad range of topics, including sexuality. The deeper feelings related to sex are not easily surveyed. No matter how large a sample is used in the most comprehensive study, it cannot give a heart's view or capture how men experience their sexuality in the secret recesses of their psyches. An in-depth interview is needed to do this. Ongoing, long-term psychotherapy is about the best in-depth technique I know.

Second, for the past sixteen years or so I have taught classes in the doctor of ministry program of the seminary where I serve as dean of the school of psychology. I have taught this class to more than six hundred clergy, most of them men. As a part of this class each student is required to provide me with a confidential paper that forthrightly addresses personal issues including their struggles with sexuality. While I treat this information with the utmost confidentiality, it has provided me with incomparable information about how men with high moral values experience their sexuality.

Third, in order to obtain an appropriate and objective database, a thorough, candid questionnaire was constructed addressing the subject matter found in the following chapters. At the time of writing this report, six hundred responses have been analyzed. This analysis provides objective data on how men feel about sex. Together, all three sources of data give me a very clear picture of how ordinary, mainstream men handle their sexuality.

By design, I have used a select sample of men. It does not in any way represent the general male population. It samples males who, by and large, consider themselves to be religious and of high moral standards. I suppose one could say that the sample represents the sexually conservative end of the male spectrum. Many of the men studied are Protestant clergy. Others come from a wide variety of occupations but have strong church connections. In analyzing this limited sample, I have tried to monitor the internal consistency of the findings to see whether there is a lot of variation. It appears, however, that the sample shows a great degree of consistency. There is not a lot of variability in this group of men.

The main advantage in studying this select group is that it helps to understand the sexual experience and struggles of those who try to live a more moral lifestyle. It paints a picture of one end of the male spectrum. To put it in a nutshell: *This is as good as it gets*. Whether their experience is healthy or not we will determine as we go. Some of it is. Some of it isn't.

For the record, the mean age of my sample is forty-one years, with a standard deviation of ten (the measure of degree of spread). Their ages ranged from seventeen to seventy-two. The vast majority were in the thirty- to fifty-year age group. Their marital status is as depicted in Figure 1.1.

Fourth, the final data I will incorporate into this report are those that come from the larger, well-known studies already done. Wherever necessary, I will draw on them for information. While these studies are generally too broad-based for my liking, the statistics they provide, when screened for bias and properly interpreted, can provide supplementary data to those I provide. There's no point in reinventing the whole wheel.

Using these four sources of information, then, I hope to be able to present a clear report of how good men experience their sexuality. For some it will be a disappointing picture. If these men are so good, how come they

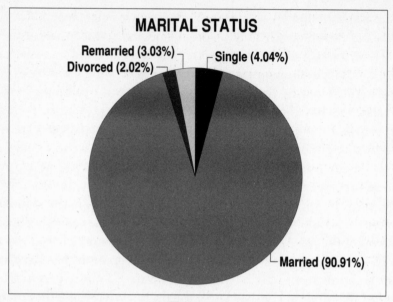

MARITAL STATUS

Remarried (3.03%)
Divorced (2.02%)
Single (4.04%)
Married (90.91%)

Figure 1.1

have so many problems? But for most of us, it is a relief to discover that we're not as off-base as we feared we were.

Background to This Report

How does this report differ from those of other researchers or theorists? Ever since Freud helped us to accept sexuality as a basic aspect of human existence we've been trying to grasp its depths and measure its heights. Freud's contribution to our understanding of sexuality, derived mainly from his therapy with patients, lies mainly in helping us understand the realm of repression. Sexuality has tremendous power to create guilt and shame; many people repress their sexuality to avoid these feelings.

Freud taught us that an unhealthy sexual exposure and activity in childhood can lead to repression of these events. This leads to maladjustments and emotional difficulties in adulthood. Today we appreciate these insights as we uncover how much childhood sexual abuse there is all around us.

But it wasn't until the post–World War II years that the first major survey of human sexual behavior was undertaken by Alfred C. Kinsey, a zoologist, and his research team. They published two volumes of findings on human sexuality, *Sexual Behavior in the Human Male*[1] (1948) and *Sexual Behavior in the Human Female*[2] (1953).

These reports should have been the final word on the matter of human sexuality, but due to faulty research techniques and sampling, several of Kinsey's conclusions are still being questioned. Some people even believe he had a radical personal agenda aimed at giving moral validation to sexual practices that the civilized world has always regarded as unnatural. Particularly contentious were his work and reports on childhood orgasm and the apparent bias against females.

Kinsey's team either didn't understand or understated the evidence of harm done to girls who are the victims of sexual abuse. Today we know differently. Adult sexual contact with children, boys *and* girls, is not a source of pleasure but frequently the source of severe emotional trauma in adulthood.[3]

Rather than helping normal or average males understand their sexuality, Kinsey only muddied the waters further. He pushed the boundaries further than a reasonable interpretation of his data could allow and introduced too many radical ideas. He even advocated "cross-generational sex," a label that was introduced to reduce the shock impact of what more accurately should be labeled sex between adults and children. He also used a high percentage of either sexual offenders or prisoners to reflect the average male's experience of sexuality. So much for Kinsey!

The next major research project was that of William Masters (a gynecologist) and his research assistant, Virginia Johnson. Their work, *Human Sexual Response*, was published in 1966 and focused mainly on the physiology of sexual arousal and orgasmic response, especially of women.[4] The techniques they developed became the basis of their sexual therapy.

No doubt, their techniques helped many to achieve a healthier sexual expression or overcome serious sexual dysfunction. But their work did nothing to expand our understanding of the inner sexual world of the male. There is more to be known about the male sexual response than technique or methods of arousal. There are feelings, inner struggles with inappropriate sexual excitement, containment of sexual feelings, and the experience of sexual frustration and anger when sexually deprived. There is also that deviousness that can only be described by the old-fashioned word *lust*. Masters and Johnson had nothing to say about these deeper concerns.

For a long time following Masters and Johnson's *Human Sexual Response*, the male was ignored. Several books emerged that tried to help. These included Barry McCarthy's *What You Still Don't Know about Male Sexuality*[5] (1977), Bernie Zilbergeld's *Male Sexuality*[6] (1978), and Herb Goldberg's *The New Male*[7] (1979).

But it wasn't until 1993 that a major revision of everything we know about sexual behavior appeared in the form of *The Janus Report on Sexual Behavior*.[8] Forty-five years after Kinsey, after interviewing nearly eight thousand Americans over nine years, Samuel and Cynthia Janus purported to give us a more accurate picture of American sexual behaviors than Kinsey. While assuring us that their sample cut across social classes and geographical boundaries, they presented some startling findings.

For instance, they say sexual activity among eighteen- to twenty-six-year-old Americans has increased sharply over the past three years despite the AIDS epidemic. They also allege that "very religious" people actually cheat on their spouses more often than less religious people. Furthermore, they assert that conservatives (politically speaking, that is) fool around more than liberals.

I can't comment on this latter point, but since I move a lot in so-called religious circles and know a lot about the private lives of male clergy, I doubt whether the generalization that very religious people cheat more is valid. For one thing, how did they measure "very religious"? Do they mean super-fundamentalists? Did they separate out sexual practices that someone may have had before having a religious conversion from sexual behaviors after becoming very religious?

Aside from these and other paradoxes that have not been adequately explained, there is a lot of very useful information in *The Janus Report*. I will use some of their data to confirm or question my own understanding of normal male sexuality.

In Search of Deeper Understanding

As we take a closer look at male sexuality, I hope to help the normal, mainstream man understand and integrate his sexuality into the rest of his being. And the women who read this book can participate in that process—a loving understanding of a man's sexual needs and conflicts can go a long way toward building a strong, satisfying relationship. Sex, after all, is the most intimate form of human communication we know between the sexes, but it has its own language and expression. Unfortunately, men and women often speak different sexual languages, and this can spell trouble for a marriage.

To men I would be quick to say: There is more to sex than knowing the erogenous zones and being a good technician at lovemaking. A good lover doesn't shy away from real intimacy and deep sharing. Once he understands his sexuality, a man can invoke and maintain feelings of tenderness and closeness far beyond the bedroom.

The male sex drive is a powerful force that can easily go off the rails of normalcy. Perversions are all around us. This is neither a fix-it book or a how-to manual. But my message is that we can control and focus our sexual energy in a healthy manner. We can reduce the tendency toward compulsiveness. We can moderate the urgency that dominates the sex drive.

Wives will particularly find help here in understanding their husbands. By being able to accept their spouse's strong urges, they will build the greatest protection possible against sexual failure in their own marriage. I have yet to meet a wife—accepting and nonjudgmental toward her spouse's sexuality, sharing open sexual communication with him— who had to contend with a wayward husband. Total openness in the arena of sexuality is the best protection I know against adultery.

Yes, uncontrolled sexual desire is destructive. But, as we will see, sexual flames can be controlled without complete dousing. After all, who would dare say that an appealing fire on a cold winter's night, contained in the hearth of one's home, isn't a matchless, marvelous blessing?

MALE SEXUALITY QUIZ

Myths, misconceptions, and misinformation about male sexuality abound. Many people are embarrassed to admit how little they really know. Here is a quiz to test your knowledge about male sexuality. Don't be surprised if you get many of the answers wrong. You're in good company, because many studies have shown that the average American knows little about sexuality in general and even less about the male sexual response. Answer True or False to the following questions.

1. The earliest age at which the average male adolescent first has sexual intercourse is fourteen.   T or F

2. Impotence, or difficulty sustaining an erection, is always psychological in origin.   T or F

3. Sexual desire and sexual activity in the male often extend well into old age.   T or F

4. A man's failure to achieve orgasm is a sign of dysfunction.   T or F

5. When a man experiences an erection while sleeping it is because he is having an erotic dream.   T or F

6. There is no food or drink that is especially effective as an aphrodisiac.   T or F

7. Sex the night before a sports event will drain an athlete's energy.   T or F

8. A man can reach orgasm without ejaculating.   T or F

9. Sexual intercourse is dangerous for a man who has had a heart attack.   T or F

ANSWERS

1. FALSE. Some start as early as eleven. Generally, though it is between fourteen and seventeen.

2. FALSE. Many physical reasons can cause impotence, including hardening of the penis arteries, disease, and hormonal deficiencies.

3. TRUE. Many elderly people report strong sexual interests in old age.

4. FALSE. Often psychological reasons (guilt) may inhibit orgasm, but so can temporary stress in normal men.

5. FALSE. Reflex circuits, such as when the bladder is full, can cause nocturnal erections.

6. TRUE. Forget about trying to find an aphrodisiac. The best love-producer is old-fashioned caring and tenderness.

7. FALSE. No evidence supports this belief. Sex serves many functions, but normal sex does not drain energy.

8. TRUE. In older men or men with physical weaknesses, the ejaculant goes into the bladder due to the valves not working properly. There is nothing wrong with this unless the man and his wife are trying to conceive.

9. TRUE AND FALSE. Men have been known to have heart attacks during sex, but also during sleep! Sex is no more risky than mild exercise, but men should get treatment anyway for any heart problem.

2

Am I Normal?

It was a touching letter. Tears flooded my eyes as I read it. I wasn't sure whether to feel pity for the writer's plight or anger at those who, in earlier years, contributed to his pain. Let's call him Glenn. In his mid-forties, he was an associate pastor at a large church. He had once taken a class from me that focused on issues of emotional and personal health in the ministry. That class had built enough rapport between us so that Glenn felt he could turn to me. Out of his anguish over his sexuality, he wrote:

> I can't begin to tell you how bothered I am by my sexual feelings. Not that my feelings don't give me pleasure—they do. In fact, I wonder sometimes whether I get more pleasure out of sex than the average male. I don't know. This is not something men in my circles talk about. In fact, I don't think men anywhere talk about the deep issues of sex. They're too ashamed or embarrassed or whatever. But if I were to boil my problem down to one question it would be this: AM I NORMAL? Almost anything can turn me on, not just my wife. A woman's smile, the flash of nudity on TV, my own thoughts, a sexual joke, or even animals doing it. I think about sex all the time or at least it feels like all the time.

What's wrong with me? AM I NORMAL? Why do I feel so much guilt about sex? Is it possible that there's a connection between the guilt that was ingrained in me as a child and the way I feel about sex now?

A long letter it was. It traced some of Glenn's early development, how he was reprimanded as a little child for touching his genitals in the bathtub. It is not uncommon for a little boy to be enamored with his penis. But Glenn's parents' excessive concern made him even more fascinated. At first, when he was only three, Glenn made no sexual connections with his touching. However, in the years that followed, the connection strengthened and flooded his consciousness. A mixture of guilt and pleasure associated with self-stimulation became fixed in his little mind. Today his mind is not so little. Nor is his problem.

There clearly is a connection between early rigid guilt (also known as false guilt) and excessive sexual preoccupation, and I will explore this later. For now, let me focus on Glenn's pleading question, a question I believe many men ask themselves from time to time: AM I NORMAL?

What Is Normal?

While undertaking the research that forms the basis for this book, I received letters from several men who questioned the whole idea of normal sexuality. In fact, any attempt these days to try defining normalcy in the realm of sexuality is usually met with a great degree of skepticism, if not downright ridicule. The argument goes something like this:

- Men are all created differently. How can you take any group of men and say that their experience is normal?

- Each man's own sexual development is different; family and school instruction about sexuality differs greatly from man to man.

- Men are exposed to pornography in different ways and at different times, causing different effects from man to man.

- Men differ in personal energy, basic personality, and sexual desire, so how can anything be normal?

These concerns are all very sound, and there is some truth to them. But they miss my point. By the term *normal*, I am not implying that male sexuality ought to fall into simple categories of normal and abnormal or within a narrow band of feelings and behavior where only one expression is healthy or acceptable.

There are many ways to understand the concept of normal. The most common way is statistical. Just count the number of men who do this or that, compute the averages, and you have what is normal. Here normal is defined merely by what the majority does or does not do. But just because everyone is doing it doesn't make something normal. It just makes it common.

If every male in a given country, for instance, has decayed teeth, you still couldn't conclude that it is normal to have bad teeth. On the other hand, you cannot ignore what is common or experienced by the majority either. You can't claim that normal is having a perfect set of teeth. Too few have perfect teeth for this to be normal, and it would exclude men with slight defects or dentures. Normal is not the same as desirable.

Both the common experience and the content, or outcome, must be taken into account in trying to define what is normal.

Finding out what is common is a good starting point in studying sexuality. But we must also ask *content* questions of ourselves, questions like: Is it healthy? Is it free of harm? Is it desirable?

If something is common and healthy, then it is probably normal as well, in the sense that I will use the word.

In the study and research that underlies this book, my starting point was first to determine what is common to the experience of good men. I need to know how many men do this or feel that. Then I apply the content questions: "Is it desirable?" or "Is it healthy?"

Obviously there are many differences between men, and being different doesn't make us abnormal. The problem is, too many men feel abnormal just because they fear or imagine that they are different. I hope my study will show that much of what every male feels and experiences is very common. Whether or not it is desirable will have to be determined by looking at its long-term effects.

As I report on my findings and try to interpret the findings of other researchers, I will apply certain content questions. I happen to have a morality that is Judeo-Christian, and this will influence my content questions and interpretations. I do not apologize for this; I believe that the vast majority of men out there are concerned about the same issues I am.

Why is the question of normalcy so important, however? The presence, direction, and intensity of the sexual drive at any given moment defines who we are as men. The nature of our sexuality determines whether we are good men or bad, healthy or neurotic, love-filled or hateful. Sexuality can shape our fathering ability and enable us to nurture, build intimacy, and maintain our successful marriages.

The man who just accepts his base sexuality for what it is and has no desire to purify any contamination within himself is robbing himself of an opportunity to really grow up. He will struggle through life carrying unnecessary baggage. He will be an incomplete man.

Why Do Men Wonder If They Are Normal?

These are not easy times for men. Their world is changing rapidly, and men are left to wallow in a confused sea of change without any clear direction. Our culture is morally confused, and this is affecting us all. We are not only puzzled about what normal is in regard to our sexuality, but about what it means to be male. This explains the current interest in exploring the myths surrounding the masculine mystique.

I am not referring to the inevitable diminution of the masculine privilege or power taking place in our culture through the rightful emergence of women's rights. Nor am I talking about the vanishing autonomous male role where he could be counted on to be a strong achiever and provider in every family. I am not even alluding to the changes taking place through male liberation groups, or the freedom men are now finding in discovering their feelings and deeper needs. These are positive changes that can help all men. They certainly contribute to happier marriages, healthier children, and a better civilization.

The confusion I am referring to is in the arena of basic sexuality.

Sexual Norms in History

We cannot fully understand why so many men ask themselves the question "Am I normal?" without a brief look at our history. Men and women were not always physically able to enjoy sex.[1] In late-seventeenth-century England, for instance, sickness, poor sanitation, and filth made sex a dangerous practice. People suffered from syphilis, crippling illness, bad breath (no dentists or disinfectants in those days), ulcers, and skin lesions. Without antibiotics, nearly all women suffered repeated vaginal and urinary-tract infections that made sex painful.

Not a pretty picture. Forget about those misleading romantic historical novels—they are fantasies. In those days, sex was not as glamorous and pleasurable as it looks in today's movies. It was often brutal, taken by force by unfeeling husbands in a world that provided little legal protection for the female. By today's standards such activity would almost invariably be labeled rape. Even the rich upper classes had to resort to excessive powdering and to wearing little bottles of incense or perfume under the nose to mask body odor and bad-smelling sores. Sex was, for the majority, animalistic and far removed from intimacy. In those days people rarely thought about what was normal or not. Low sexual desire was considered to be a good thing—one lived longer by avoiding sex. Syphilis was everywhere.

The idea of what is or isn't normal, then, is very much a twentieth-century development.[2] This is why so few experts are comfortable defining it. Is it normal to have no desire for sex? Is it normal to want a lot of sex? Is it normal to be somewhere between these two extremes? Whatever the situation, many men are deeply troubled by the question of normality.

It is only in recent history that we have begun to separate sex from the fear of pregnancy. Suddenly it became okay for women to enjoy sex without the fear of pregnancy. This has put men under pressure to perform, and these days the proof of one's manhood is how he performs in bed.

Some men, bothered by their low sexual desire, literally dread going to bed. They delay the inevitable and stay glued to the TV until they drop. They lie as far away as possible from their partner, fearing that some inadvertent touch might give rise to an expectation for sex that would test their manhood. Even when they escape sex, guilty, anxious feelings disturb them. "Why am I this way? What's wrong with me? Why can't I be a real man? Am I normal?"

A larger percentage of men is found at the other end of the spectrum. But these concerned men are not perverts naked under their raincoats and waiting to expose themselves. They are respectable men in well-cut suits who hold responsible positions. They occasionally (sometimes often) masturbate by themselves just to get some relief from their pent-up

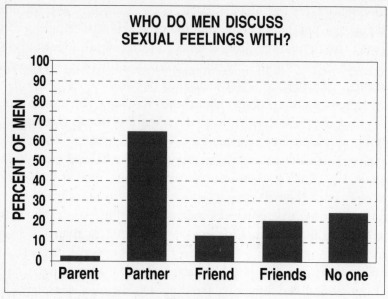

Figure 2.1

sexual tensions. Periodically they watch a risqué movie. Sex is seldom far from their minds. All of them don't go to sleazy X-rated movie houses or massage parlors or even rent X-rated videos. They stick with steamy love scenes from PG-rated movies. But they ask the same questions: "Why am I this way? What's wrong with me? Why can't I be normal?"

In cases where they're dealing with low or high levels of sexual desire, these men have no idea just how common their problems are. Both are normal. They just don't know it or won't believe it.

It's difficult for men to look to each other to discover what is normal. Who does one take as a role model? The hero in the movie? Get real! How come those silver-screen idols never have real problems? And should we look to our work buddies? They tell dirty jokes to cover up their hidden secrets but never talk seriously about sex—they're too embarrassed!

So with whom can men discuss their sexual feelings? I posed this question to my sample of men. Figure 2.1 presents the results. Very few ever discuss their sexual feelings with their parents. Parents got the lowest rating. About 14 percent of the men said they had a single friend they could talk to, while 20 percent said they had several friends. About 65 percent said their partner or spouse was the only one they could talk with, while 25 percent said they had no one.

One in four men have no one, not even a wife, they can talk with about their deepest sexual thoughts or feelings. My guess is that even those men who said they could talk with their partners would admit that there is a limit to what they can talk about. All men have deep secrets in the realm of their sexuality—hidden feelings that are created early, then pushed down. These are dark, frightening thoughts they'd never dare share because such revelations would be embarrassing beyond words. Few men ever talk about them to anyone.

What Questions Bother Men about Sexuality?

Beneath the Am I normal? question there lies a long list of more specific concerns. Different men ask the following three questions for different reasons.

Question #1: Am I oversexed?

This is the most common question I hear from healthy men. For instance, Don asked it not too long ago. We were discussing his small business, which wasn't doing so well. Don had no energy. No interest. He couldn't get himself going in the morning. He wasted hours and hours of his time just moping around or allowing himself to be distracted. Since he was his own boss, he wasn't accountable to anyone whether he worked or not.

I probed his sleeping habits. "Oh, I get to bed at one or two in the morning," he said. Why? He explained that he waited for his wife to go to bed, hoping she would invite him to have sex. When she didn't, he would watch TV for a long time, partly because he was angry but also because he was looking for some stimulation. Night after night Don sat there clicking away on the remote. He had calluses to prove it. Eventually, he would "let the TV lead me to the Playboy channel."

Don hadn't subscribed to the Playboy channel, mind you. His wife wouldn't allow it in her home. But the scrambled, fuzzy picture of people having sex intrigued him. Every now and then the picture would clear enough so that he could get a glimpse of naked bodies and hear grunting sounds. He'd feel a rush of excitement. For some reason he found an occasional glimpse of nudity more exciting than a continuous view of it. He would usually masturbate, then go to bed. Don's question was simple: Am I oversexed?

I explained to him that his problem was not one of being oversexed. However, he had created an addictive sexual taboo. (I will explain how this happens in a later chapter.) He was doing something naughty, and it was extra exciting because it was "off-limits." He needed to refocus on his sexual relationship with his wife and to break his growing dependence on the "extra" excitement he was experiencing elsewhere.

Ed asked the oversexed question for another reason. He felt he needed sex every day. He said if he didn't get it, he'd feel lousy. He couldn't settle down. He'd get restless. Ed's wife couldn't keep up with him. She had a healthy attitude about sex. She was orgasmic and enjoyed sex. And if she hadn't had to keep house, raise three small children, and keep up a part-time job to keep them financially solvent, she believed she could match Ed for sexual desire any day. But at that stage of her life, daily intercourse was out of the question. By early evening she was exhausted, and she fell asleep the moment her head hit the pillow, desire or no desire.

Ed understood, up to a point. He didn't blame his wife; he blamed himself. "Why am I so needy?" he keeps asking. "Am I oversexed?"

I sensed that he was becoming obsessive. If only we had a pill that could temporarily take away sexual desire without any other negative consequences! I gave Ed all the empathy I could muster. "Ed," I said, "you're perfectly normal. You are blessed with a wonderful, responsive wife. The problem is your stage in life. There are too many other demands on your wife to expect her to be able to match your sexual needs at this time."

I went on to suggest that we discuss other frustrations in Ed's work-life that might be causing his neediness. Often men use sexual orgasm as a form of tranquilizer or tension releaser. Furthermore, I suggested some ways he and his wife could keep sexuality within their relationship without his imposing intercourse on her. Manual stimulation, for example, could be enjoyable to both and is perfectly healthy *if it is shared together*. I finally told Ed that his obsession about being oversexed was making him more sexually self-conscious and therefore needy.

At this point I should hasten to add that not every man who complains about being oversexed is necessarily within normal limits. Since the sex drive is hormonally driven, it stands to reason that things can go wrong.

A small percentage of the male population really is beyond hormonal normalcy, and out-of-control hormones can be a serious, even dangerous, problem. If you have any doubt, see a doctor and reassure yourself that everything is working properly biologically.

For most men, however, the oversexed problem is not an abnormal hormonal system, but rather a distorted perspective. The Am I oversexed? question has more to do with the learned ways of *expressing* sexuality than with the basic mechanisms of sexual arousal. The sexual impulse is an instinct, like hunger and thirst, that demands satisfaction through the relief of a peculiar type of tension. But the excitement and pleasure that accompanies sexual activity is *mainly learned.*[3]

Question #2: Am I Undersexed?

The Am I normal? question is not only linked to oversex, but also to undersex. This question is also asked for different reasons. Jim and Connie would, by their own admission, be considered yuppies. They've been married for six years and have no children but lots of dogs, cats, cars, and debts. Both have careers. Both have their own bank accounts. And both suffer from headaches, regular bouts of the flu, and little time for sex. In fact, they are among those known as DINS—Dual Income, No Sex couples.

It wasn't always this way. When Jim and Connie first married they both loved sex and enjoyed it often. But lifestyle exhaustion slowly wore them down. They stopped putting energy into their sexuality and sent it elsewhere. Now they were on different schedules, like ships that pass in the night. Sex had moved down to a place of low priority, a virtual stranger to their relationship.

Jim was the one who woke up one day to realize what was happening. "Am I undersexed?" was his question. "Not really," I told him, "but we have fantastic minds. Our minds can be distracted and their energies redirected. Our minds can turn off the sexual machinery and keep us focused on other exciting activities. When it's healthy, we call this process *sublimation.*"

Is this normal? Of course it is. How else do celibate people sublimate their sexual energies? Their wonderful minds can take care of the problem. Can sexual desire be changed? Certainly. It's all a matter of choice. If you don't want to be bothered by sex, you find some other meaningful activity that is more captivating and rewarding, give it your all, and you can say good-bye to your sex drive.

Simple as that? Not really. I doubt if I could turn it off that easily. But apparently there are those who can. Of course, they may find that their alternative preoccupations give them more headaches, ulcers, and stress disease than sex. But the choice is there.

Nevertheless, Jim was worried. He sensed that he and Connie were drifting apart. He even suspected that she might be having casual sex outside of the marriage. Why else was she so disinterested? What if this state of affairs continued? What if he lost her to some oversexed macho male who would come charging into her life and sweep her off her feet?

I warned Jim that after replacing sexual desire with other exciting things like a career, money, and living it up there's only about a 50 percent chance of reversing the problem.[4] Jim was startled.

"It takes time," I reassured him. Soon Jim and Connie began to work on their problem together. Here was the prescription:

1. Take some time to review and reconsider your priorities. Ask yourselves: What is important in our lives?

2. Revise your value system. Why are money and success so important to us? What else should we begin to value as a couple? What about having a family?

3. Consider sacrificing some of your lifestyle. Work out compromises. You can't have your cake and eat it, too. Something must go.

4. Take time out to rediscover each other. Build your love by building your friendship.

5. Work at recapturing the pleasure of sexual feelings in general. Don't just focus on intercourse. Hold hands. Touch each other. Spend more time alone.

Men who have hormonal problems are also prone to ask the "Am I undersexed?" question. Researchers now know that sexual desire is triggered in the brain by testosterone, with the help of other "messengers" like dopamine. The mind and body form a complex chemical machine, and unless they are working normally, don't expect to feel the right amount of sexuality. Again, if you are in any doubt, have yourself checked out by a competent physician who specializes in this area.

Question #3: Can I control my sex drive?

For many men the sex drive feels like a volcano. Explosive and unpredictable, it continues to burn deep down in the groin, even when there's no reason for it. It may lay dormant for a while, only grumbling occasionally. But it awakens sooner or later, and when it erupts it spews out fiery magma uncontrollably. It can lay waste to everything in its path including honor, reputation, families, virginity, fidelity, chastity, good intentions, life-long promises, and spiritual commitments.

On one hand sexual feelings can be innocent, pure, and holy. On the other, sexuality can be savage, frenzied, hideous, and lurid.

Since the dawn of time, the vicious nature of male sexuality has been responsible for the most terrible crimes against children, women, and other men. Jeffrey Dahmer didn't ravish, debauch, and dismember his victims just for entertainment or because he was bored. He didn't victimize and brutalize his captives just to vent his rage at humanity or to experiment with his power over people. He did it for sexual gratification, plain and simple. He was driven by his sick need for a certain form of sexual gratification.

The same has been true of scores of other serial killers, rapists, and child abusers who, interestingly, are almost always males. This clearly indicates that the male sex drive can be a very destructive force when it goes off the rails of normalcy. The gratification of the sexual instinct has the potential to exemplify the worst in human evil. It can reduce the most sophisticated male to the level of the brute beast of the jungle. Not a pretty picture. But it is reality.

So it is in this context that I hear men asking: Can I control my sex drive? Are all the men who struggle to understand and control their "sexual beast within," weirdos, crackpots, or deranged sociopaths? Definitely not! They are average, well-brought-up, and generally healthy. But their volcano is not extinct, either, and they know it is merely waiting for a moment of weakness before it erupts.

Why Is Control Necessary?

Every male transitioning from childhood through adolescence to adulthood has to develop a system of self-control over his sexuality. It is alarming how few parents understand this. Many believe it just happens—leave it alone and it will take care of itself. True? Not at all. And what happens when it doesn't?

It's interesting to note that in less westernized cultures, sexual intercourse is not the highly secretive activity it is for us. Nudity is not a source of shame, and sexual instruction of the young is as natural and spontaneous as it appears to be in primates. In general, sexuality in these settings is without the neurotic features that characterize it in Western culture today.

So far so good!

But this is not the whole picture. These cultures can also be savage. Women are usually the common property of men and the spoil of conquest. Viewed as chattel, women are considered to be articles of commerce. They can be traded, bartered, and possessed, as well as abused and cast aside when expended. Whenever attitudes and practices like this prevail, there is little need to control sexuality. Men get whatever they want and do whatever they want. Such a behavior can hardly be labeled as *civilized*. It is beastly and abusive.

A long time ago a revolution occurred to change this. It came in the form of religion, or Christianity to be precise.[5] The promotion of a more refined development of sexual life followed, when women ceased to be viewed as property. Raising the status of women did not take away the need for sexual control. In fact, it increased it. Moral imperatives had to counteract hormonal imperatives. Men could not just follow the urge of their raging desires. The equation is simple: For women to be free, sexuality has to be contained.

So the apostle Paul wrote: "that each of you should learn to control his own body in a way that is holy and honorable" (1 Thess. 4:4 NIV).

Thanks to Christianity, monogamy became the law in the Western world, the norm in both religious and social systems. Wherever Christianity went, women were liberated and their status was elevated so that they began to be viewed as socially equal to men. Meanwhile, alongside this liberation the sexuality of the male also had to be contained and confined. This made stable and long-term relationships possible.

Compare, if you will, those cultures that were influenced by Christianity with those that were not. The status of women is the touchstone. Many non-Christian cultures still bar women from public life, grant the right of divorce only to men, stifle female intellectual development, and view women as male possessions. Under such conditions women are seen to be nothing more than a means for sexual gratification and the propagation of the race. And always accompanying such oppressive cultural patterns, freedom of sexual expression is granted to the male, often without any legal or social consequences.

The oppression of women and the lack of control of male sexual expression have always been linked together. You don't see one without the other. If women are to be free, then men must control their sexual urges. For men to have unrestrained sexual privileges, women must be in some form of bondage. If sexuality is to be extravagant in a culture, women must be compliantly oppressed.

Yet in today's society, we are rapidly reverting to an uncontrolled sexuality. A widely accepted "free-sex" philosophy, in which commitment is not seen by males to be a prerequisite for sexual expression, is rampant. Free sex is once again turning women into chattel, only at the moment many of them don't seem to see it. Women are being pressured to satisfy men's sexual needs in order to win favor or find a marriage partner. This amounts to another form of enslavement. Ultimately all women must be the losers if the idea that free sex, with no need for commitment, continues out of control.

Already we are seeing dramatic changes in masculine attitudes to commitment. Men want full sexual privileges without any obligations, least of all that of marriage. A significant majority of men today appear to be able to satisfy their sexual needs without resorting to or having a need for stable relationships. Fly-by-night sex and one-night stands are the order of the day. "Why should I get married?" a male patient asked me recently. "I can get all the sex I need without any obligations." And he's right. Men no longer have any incentive to build stable, long-term marital relationships. It appears that in today's world, sexual expression is no longer something people think we need to control. And the losers, once again, are women.

A Glimmer of Hope

Am I painting too pessimistic a picture of the current state of affairs regarding male sexuality? If so, allow me to end this chapter with a few positive comments.

Many young adults today are concerned about what is happening to their sexuality. They are beginning to consider the dangers of pornography and are weighing whether or not intercourse before marriage is really such a good idea after all.

Also, the kids of baby boomers are learning valuable lessons from their parents. Men and women who grew up in the 1960s and 1970s saw it all. They were part of the sexual revolution and the emergence of the drug culture, but they don't want their children to make the same mistakes they did. Days of rage and nights of pleasure have left them fully aware of the hazards of misguided morals. These parents are willing to have frank, open discussions about sex—the kind of conversations all parents are supposed to have with their children.

These parents don't want to create a repressive environment like the ones they rebelled against, but they also seem to be saying, "Start the revolution without my kid." They want their sons and daughters to say no to inappropriate sex. They don't want them to have to go for abortions; better they shouldn't get pregnant in the first place. These men and women realize that kids growing up today are playing with high stakes. Wrong sex can kill you. AIDS is no joke, and condoms are not a foolproof protection.

Above all, baby boomers can speak with authority. They can tell their own horror stories about promiscuous sex, knowing all too well that the choices made today have consequences tomorrow. They can say with great integrity, "We were foolish and made a lot of mistakes Don't make the same mistakes we did." No double messages. No judgment. No rejection. Just plain, old-fashioned honesty.

Three cheers for such parents! They are not only going to produce healthier children, but their daughters will be protected from exploitation. And their sons won't grow up constantly asking the question, Am I normal?

HOW WELL DO YOU UNDERSTAND MALE SEXUALITY?

Read the following statements and decide whether you believe them to be true or false.

1. More men than women have experienced unwanted intercourse. T or F

2. More "very religious" men cheat on their wives than nonreligious men. T or F

3. Just as fat in the bloodstream can block arteries in the heart, so it starts to block arteries in the penis preventing adequate erection. T or F

4. Men also experience a male menopause. T or F

5. After marriage most men stop masturbating. T or F

6. According to most sex therapists, what most men complain about is not getting enough oral sex. T or F

7. Getting married remedies all the problems men have with lust. T or F

8. Boys who are sexually repressed while growing up are more likely to become obsessed with masturbation and pornography when they are grown up. T or F

Choose which answer you believe is most correct for the following:

9. How often does the average, healthy male think about sex?
(a) once a month, (b) once a week, (c) once a day, (d) once an hour

10. How many men would complain that they don't get enough sex?
(a) 20%, (b) 35%, (c) 50%, (d) 70%

11. The average age at which the American male first has sex is
(a) 14, (b) 16, (c) 18, (d) 20

12. Where does the average young male learn most about sex?
(a) From the home, (b) from friends, (c) from books, (d) from pornography.

ANSWERS

1. TRUE. Contrary to what most people think, more men say they have felt forced into unwanted sex either to prove themselves or to comply with peer pressure.

2. TRUE. *The Janus Report* provides data to support the idea that "very religious" men are at greater risk for cheating than "just religious" men. It could well be that they repress their sexuality more and thus do not acknowledge their true sexual feelings.

3. TRUE. The same cholesterol that blocks heart arteries can shut off blood to the penis and inhibit full erections. (Reference: *Men's Health*, Sept./Oct. 1992, 42)

4. FALSE. Men do not experience menopause (another myth). While hormones decline gradually, the majority of men remain sexually active into their seventies, eighties, or beyond. Frequency does decline, however.

5. FALSE. Many men may at first reduce the frequency of their masturbation, but return to it later. Those men that learn during adolescence how to masturbate to pornography find it difficult to break the habit later.

6. TRUE. Men in our culture easily become obsessed with oral sex—giving it and receiving it. No satisfactory theory for this has yet been put forward; most experts believe it is not abnormal. However, some health risks do exist and many women find it repugnant!

7. FALSE. When men get married, lust does not subside. Men have to learn how to redirect their arousal back to their appropriate partners. Lust, when uncontrolled, creates many unpleasant situations including inappropriate sexual harassment.

8. TRUE. A sexually repressive upbringing creates excessive guilt around sexual feelings and this sets up the obsessive need for masturbation.

9. D. Most men think about sex at least several times a day or an hour. Younger men, under age thirty-five, think about it even more often. Interestingly, after age thirty-five the frequency remains about the same.

10. D. According to other major studies 70 percent of men complain that they don't get enough sex. Interestingly, 58 percent of women make the same complaint. In my study 28 percent of married men said their needs were not adequately met.

11. B. The average American male has his first sexual encounter at age sixteen. However, 20 percent report that they had their first sexual relations before the age of fourteen. There is strong evidence that the age of puberty continues to drop, so more and more men are now reporting first sexual encounters at the age of eleven or earlier.

12. D. Most young males have their sexual beliefs and attitudes shaped by pornography. Exposure often begins at age thirteen. This distorts their views of how women feel about sex and what can reasonably be expected from sex, and it sets them up for disappointment in the real world. Real women cannot possibly measure up to the air-brushed, color-enhanced, glossy photographs that become the standard of reference for most males.

3

Why Male Sexuality
Goes Wrong

Male sexuality is not in a healthy place, and it's not just because men don't get enough sex. There are also problems inherent in the ways men want their erotic needs met. For a number of reasons, male sexuality has taken a detour, heading in several wrong directions. Many men have lost their way.

I see male sexuality by and large as neurotic. It has become obsessional—it dominates too much thinking—and compulsive—it engages in behaviors that are irresistible and lack control. Men use sex for more than just sexual gratification. And as I've said before, I'm talking here about good, heterosexual men whose behavior is discreet and respectful of others.

Sex has become taboo in our society.[1] It is unmentionable, especially in the company of good people. Some parents talk to their kids about it in terms of birds, bees, and flowers. In hopes that the kids will lose interest in it, they avoid plain facts. And even when the facts are forthrightly addressed, many of us avoid talking about the feelings of sex: its force, urgency, overwhelming preoccupation, and the "let down" that follows when it is satisfied.

Children also have to learn from their own feelings what sexuality is all about. And if we haven't learned to discuss sexual matters openly, how can we tell if others feel the same way we do? How can we know whether

35

our feelings are normal? We can't. So we become confused and join millions of other males in their confusion.

Sex is an excessively secret thing, involving too much intrigue and mystery. When anything is secretive, it has the potential to become distorted and even neurotic. It is in the soil of concealment that seeds of sexual addiction, anxiety, depression, compulsions, phobias, and dissociations are planted.

Male Sexuality—Simple or Complex?

There is a widely held myth in our culture that men are very simple creatures when it comes to sex.[2] Supposedly, men have no special requirements. The "equipment" for sex is straightforward, always ready for use, and easy to satisfy. Male sexuality is not cluttered with a complex need for tenderness, intimate communication, or preparation ritual. Foreplay is not viewed as a male need, just a female need.

According to this myth, men are ready to perform sexually at the drop of a hat (or anything else). They have simple tastes but insatiable appetites, and they tremble in terror at only two threats: impotence and having to share their feelings. If men had their way they would divorce sex from love, including gentleness and cuddling. They only put up with these inconveniences in order to get the sex they desperately need.

Above all, says the myth, men never have any doubts or questions about sex. There is no confusion. Men know how they compare with other men because they all talk openly about their desires and achievements. Males know all there is to know about how to have good sex.

True? Absolutely not. Contrary to these myths and stereotypes, men are confused. They are worried. Males are mostly extremely secretive about their inner sexual feelings and experiences; they rarely talk about them. Consequently, they have no idea how their feelings and experiences compare with those of other men.

Almost every man tends to think that he is the only one with problems—everyone else is having a great time. Only he has to put up with an experience that is less than what he would like it to be. He keeps his mouth shut, fakes it, and pretends to be confident and comfortable. Every male I know wonders whether he's missing out on something.

Male sexuality is not simple at all. In fact, it is highly complex. Men learn their sexuality haphazardly, by trial and error. For every healthy male, life is a never-ceasing duel between the animal instinct (some call it the "flesh"), and morality. Sexual inclinations push the boundaries of decency and test the moral fibers of the clearest, straightest, and most honorable men I know.

One of the reasons why sex is complex for the male is because his ego gets so wrapped up in it. Every male who has ever lived has, at some time or another, worried about his dimensions or erectile strength—if not his size, then his prowess. Real men last forever, real men are big, they think. So, I can't be a real man can I? Of course both statements are untrue, but they linger in the male mind anyway.

Unlike many women, men aren't comfortable talking about sex because it puts their egos on the line, revealing deep, dark secrets. We sometimes accuse men of having no feelings just because they can't express them. But they do have feelings—lots of them. Unfortunately, they aren't at all comfortable revealing them either to men or to women.

Growing up among other boys, males have to brag and posture. They don't survive otherwise. When grown, they observe a code of silence about their sexual exploits, which often amount to more dreams and failures than to successes. In our culture, inexpressiveness in men is shaped just as surely as femininity in girls. Both mothers and father are sometimes guilty of stifling male emotional expression as unmanly or effeminate.

There is a further problem. As Zilbergeld explains, our culture tends to label any positive feelings men have toward one another as sexual.[3] Tenderness, for the male, becomes synonymous with sexuality. Physical affection is one of the faces of sex. Why do many men feel awkward hugging other men? Because they fear it could be perceived as sexual. So tenderness, the desire to be with someone, and physical touching become taboo. As we noted before, this even damages the relationships between father and daughters.

Sex is also complex for the male because of another key issue—he does not really see sex as linked to love. This is such a fundamental difference from the way women see sex that you really wonder how men and women ever get together on this issue. In my sexual survey I asked men to answer yes or no to the statement, "I believe it is physically possible to have sex with someone I don't love." The overwhelming majority of men responded yes. In fact, 81 percent of them answered affirmatively.

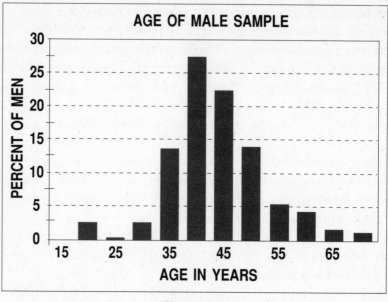

Figure 3.1

I don't ever recall a female patient who would agree with this. Love and sex are inextricably linked in most women's thinking. Not so for men. And remember, the respondents to my sexual survey were good men, most of them deeply Christian and committed to a high moral system. Of course, they didn't say they would have sex with someone they didn't love, only that they could. Several wrote me notes to emphasize this point. Being honest about your feelings is not the same as committing the act.

This is why platonic love or friendship can be so easily misread by males. A woman, for instance, might think that only a friendship is developing, perhaps with a male acquaintance at work. She enjoys doing things with him. She knows the boundaries. They laugh, share stories, and have lunch. For her it is all platonic, pure friendship. There's no love, so there can't possibly be anything sexual, assuming she's not trying to seduce him in the hope that the relationship will go further.

The man, oblivious to his deeper feelings, only thinks with his hormones. "She's interested in sex," he thinks. "She's got to be. Why else would she be so friendly?" Is he right? Not at all. And if he tries to take it further, he could be in serious trouble.

Men and women view the link between love and sex differently. But instead of making sex simpler for men, this difference makes it more complex.

Men don't have an innate defense against sexual arousal, so they have to construct it for themselves. Not many men are effective in creating this protection, so ladies beware. Men don't always do a good job of being "just friends" with a woman.

The Beginnings of Male Sexuality

The starting point in my study examined the beginnings of men's sexuality. It has revealed some interesting facts. Figure 3.1 presents the age distribution of the sample. These men represent a fairly stable group of married men. Their ages ranged from seventeen to over seventy and those who were married had been married for an average of 15.1 years. Here are some of the questions I wanted answered.

At what age do men first experience sexual feelings? The answer? At about 11 years of age. The average ranged from 10.71 years to 11.26 years, a very close variation through all my subgroups. A few men reported having had sexual feelings as early as 1 or 2 years of age, but very few fell into this early group. Some spoke of the awakenings of sexual feelings between 5 and 7 (see Figure 4.1 in chapter 4.) It appears that a small group of men peaked at this age then flattened in their sexual feelings before the real onslaught at 12 or 13.

The first feelings of sexuality seemed to precede the onset of puberty by about two years. The age of the onset of puberty varied from a minimum of 7 (two men reported this) to a maximum of 19. Most were in the range of 11 to 14 with the average ranging from 12.35 to 13.10 years. (See Figure 3.2.)

When do boys start to masturbate? This question will be discussed in more detail in chapter 4, but a few preliminary remarks are appropriate here. It is quite clear that some boys start masturbating before they reach the age of puberty. Between 25 percent and 30 percent of boys (an average 29 percent for the whole sample) started masturbating before they reported having reached puberty. About 5 percent reported that they did not start masturbating as teenagers, and this is consistent across all age subgroups.

The range of ages for starting to masturbate differs quite widely from a low of 7 to between 26 and 40 years of age. The average varies between

13.6 and 14.3. So we can safely say that the majority of boys start masturbating at 14, which is about one year after the average age for reaching puberty.

How frequently do boys masturbate? Because there was likely to be a difference associated with the onset of puberty, I chose to set a reference point. I asked the men how often they estimated they were masturbating per month at age sixteen, assuming, of course, that most would be masturbating by this age. Excluding those who said that they were not masturbating at this age, the average was 13.3 times per month. The range varied widely, from once a month to as many as 100 times a month. More than a quarter (27 percent) of the men reported that at age sixteen they were not masturbating. They had either never started or had stopped before this age.

How does exposure to pornographic magazines or X-rated movies affect male sexuality? This is a topic I will explore in greater depth later. Here I mainly want to comment on how early boys confront this kind of sexual exposure. The average age of introduction to pornographic materials in my sample was 15.5 years of age, just one and a half years after starting to masturbate and two and a half years after puberty. My sample showed that 7.5 percent had never been exposed to X-rated or pornographic material. The range of ages for first exposure varied from a minimum of five to a maximum of thirty-eight.

How do men feel now about the effect of this early exposure on their sexual development? Of those exposed, 62 percent reported it was destructive. Only 1.2 percent reported it was beneficial. The exposure was neutral for 32 percent in its effects upon them. The remaining men had no opinions on the matter. Those who say it was beneficial are very much in the minority. Two out of three males believe it was damaging in some way.

How healthy was the instruction in sexuality these men received growing up? The men were asked to circle all that applied in the following categories: (1) healthy/unhealthy, (2) adequate/inadequate, (3) helpful/unhelpful, (4) accurate/distorted. They were free to define these terms for themselves. I was not at all surprised by the results. More than three out of four (78 percent) reported that their instruction in sexuality while growing up was inadequate. Only 37 percent said it was healthy, and only 30 percent said it was accurate. This means that nearly three out of four men believe that their sexual instruction as children was not even correct!

I will have a lot more to say later about this portrait of sexuality. But the facts as I have presented them thus far describe a bleak beginning to male sexuality. The picture is one of early development of sexual feelings, early puberty, and early masturbation and exposure to pornography. Besides concluding that the pornography was destructive, the majority of men reported that their childhood sexual instruction was hopelessly inadequate. Not a good start. No wonder men don't finish well.

TEN UNSOLVED MYSTERIES ABOUT MALE SEXUALITY

What is it about male sexuality that is so confusing? Here are the top ten unsolved mysteries about male sexuality I have collected over the years. I hope the answers will emerge in the pages that follow.

1. Why are men so different from women in their sexuality? They respond to different stimuli, enjoy different experiences, and develop quite different sexual hang-ups.

2. Why are men more prone to develop sexual fetishes about the female body? One man focuses on one part of the female anatomy as a source of stimulation; another focuses on something else. In fact, why are men more prone than women to develop fetishes at all?

3. Why do men develop their sexual peak in the late teens or early twenties while women only reach their peak in their forties? Nature seems to have played a cruel joke on men and women.

4. Why do more men than women become more prone to linking adrenaline arousal with sex? This sometimes leads to a linking of pain with pleasure.

5. Why are men able to enjoy sex without emotions? They are also able, more so than women, to divorce the sexual act from its romantic underpinnings, a feat most women find impossible.

6. Why do men rank quantity over quality in sexual experience? Is it purely a matter of satisfying forceful hormones, or is there a deeper, more psychological reason?

7. Why do men tend to label any positive, friendly, or affectionate feeling toward women as sexual feelings? Does this in some way prevent intimacy in general, because they link intimacy with sexual feelings?

8. Why do men more commonly find it necessary to substitute pictures, pornography, or other visual forms of stimulation in order to become aroused? Why can't they be content with closeness, intimacy, or just plain old-fashioned love feelings to become aroused?

9. Why do men find taboo, naughty, or prohibited sexual behaviors more exciting than permissible ones? Is this just the makeup of male sexuality, or does it have its roots in early childhood experiences?

10. Why do men find it so difficult to understand how women experience sexuality? And why don't women understand male sexuality?

How Do Things Go Wrong?

There are four important background factors that I need to explain if I am going to adequately show how and why things go wrong with men's sexuality. They involve the age of puberty, prolonged sexual abstinence, the role of guilt, and the adrenaline connection. Although some of these factors may seem technical, a more complete understanding of them can help us all—men, women, fathers, and mothers—to do a better job of shaping healthy sexuality. It will also help to explain why some men get led astray, become sexual addicts, or develop other distortions of sexuality, including many of the perversions.

Age of puberty. The distribution of puberty age for my sample of men is depicted in Figure 3.2. As you will see it predominantly occurs in the twelve and thirteen age group. Each boy has a highly individualized schedule for moving from childhood to adulthood. Puberty represents an important transition point—at puberty a boy gains the physical ability to reproduce children. It results from the effects of various hormones on the brain and body.

When you think about it, doesn't it seem strange that boys (and girls) reach puberty at ages twelve or thirteen? They are only children, yet they

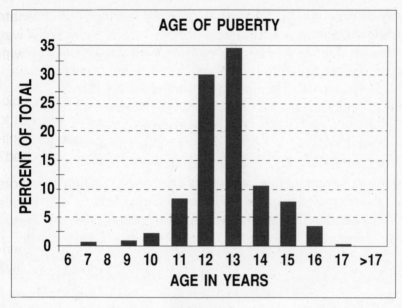

Figure 3.2

are capable of bearing children. Believe it or not, this plays a major role in determining why male sex goes wrong.

Let me address a little-realized fact about sexual development in both boys and girls. It is this: *The age of puberty is now lower than ever before in history and it continues to drop.*

Can you believe this? Just over 150 years ago, the average age of puberty in girls (and presumably also in boys) was almost 17 years. In fact, the age at which girls first menstruate has been dropping steadily for the last several centuries. In Germany the average age in 1795 was 16.6 years. By 1920 it had dropped to 14.5 years. In the United States the average age in the 1930s was 13.5, but it had dropped to below 13 by the mid 1960s.

A recent study in Nigeria compared rural boys and girls with urban boys and girls. Rural girls menstruated at a mean age of 14.54 years, whereas urban girls of the same ethnic group menstruated at a mean age of 12.67.[4]

This marked difference between urban and rural girls in their age of puberty is important. It matches the general downward trend over the last century. Why has the age of puberty dropped? Factors contributing to this drop include improved health and nutrition, more efficient healthcare, and exposure to sex-related sensual materials in magazines, television, movies, and radio.

But what about boys? Their pubertal stage is more difficult to estimate. Broken voice, nocturnal emissions, and development of pubic hair are unreliable by themselves. There are significant problems, therefore, in studies that try to determine the age of puberty. In the Nigerian study, only a small difference was found. Rural boys reach puberty around 14.7 on average, while urban boys reach it at 14.2 years. Despite the slower rate of sexual development in these boys compared to that of girls, boys too are subject to a gradual lowering of the age of puberty, corresponding to improved health and increased sexual stimulation at earlier ages.

What does this all mean? Clearly, in earlier times, puberty occurred in the late teens, possibly seventeen or eighteen years of age for both sexes. Allowing for a slightly later age of puberty for boys, this means that *the period of time between the physical readiness for sex and the age at which one could marry and experience sex was very short*. As the age of puberty has dropped, this period of waiting has increased. At the other end, the age for marriage has risen. The need for graduate education and economic readiness for starting a family can delay marriage for several years.

Generations ago, a boy reached puberty at eighteen or nineteen and could marry at twenty or twenty-one, requiring only a short waiting period before he could experience the sexuality raging within his body. Today, boys are ready at thirteen but must wait until twenty-five or even as late as thirty before they can marry, have sex in a stable relationship, and support a family. The length of time one must wait for sex has gone from one or two years to twelve to fifteen years or even longer.

Assuming that sex is reserved for a permanent relationship, it is this long period of abstinence that causes most of our problems. A thirteen-year-old boy does not have the emotional maturity to handle his sexuality. He seeks whatever outlets he can find, including promiscuous sex, masturbating to pornography, and any other sexual thrill he can find. This is the source of a great deal of distortion.

Has the age of puberty stopped dropping? Every evidence suggests not. Why should it? Health and living conditions continue to provide a perfect environment for rapid physical development. We continue to expose younger and younger children to sexual stimulation. More and more children are maturing sexually at ages eleven or twelve, some even at nine or ten. I recently read of a case where some twelve-year-old boys raped a girl. In another case, two seven-year-olds were accused of raping a six-year-old girl. How does a seven-year-old know what to do? Pregnancies are on the rise in girls under ten. It doesn't look to me like the drop is slowing down.

So what are we facing if this trend continues? Children of nine or ten are capable of having sex without the emotional maturity to handle the consequences. It is my considered opinion that we are headed for major problems in the new century. We need to study the impact distorted views and information about sexuality are having on the development of our children. If we are causing our children to become sexually promiscuous, we need to change our ways.

Prolonged sexual abstinence. Things also go wrong in male sexuality because the prolonged stage of sexual abstinence that is required of children and adolescents distorts sexuality. How does this happen? Listen to Ben's story, and realize that he is not alone in his experience.

Shortly after he had his first "wet dream" at thirteen, Ben discovered that he could masturbate. It was an overwhelming experience. At first he was totally overjoyed at the pleasure it gave him. When he discovered some *Playboy* magazines hidden in his father's cupboard, he began to view them on an almost daily basis. His heart thumped and his excitement was exhilarating as lust awakened. At thirteen, Ben's obsession with sex was formed.

For the next seven or eight years, Ben's sexuality continued on a very distorted track. *Playboy* gave way to X-rated magazines, but the pattern was always the same. Whenever he could, he collected pictures that excited him. He had a huge collection of them. The women in them became his fantasy friends. Sometimes he couldn't tell reality from fantasy. It didn't matter that "his girls" were not real.

Ben never felt guilty about what he did. No feelings of remorse. In fact, he thought everything was permissible. Unlike many of his peers, he indulged himself quite freely. But he never told anyone. He kept it private. He didn't know what other boys were doing about their sex drive, and he didn't care. It was sufficient that he was thrilled with what he experienced.

Ben occasionally tried to date girls. Not believing himself to be very attractive, he fumbled most of the time and felt he came across like a jerk. Besides, real girls didn't match the quality of his pictures. So Ben wasn't worried, even though he believed himself to be the only virgin in his high school class.

It wasn't until he got to college that Ben began to realize that he had developed a major problem with pornography. He began to call it a fixation because it gave him his "fix" whenever he was down. It gave him comfort when he felt rejected. But as he pored over his collections he began to crave the comfort and closeness of a real person. Someone to talk to. Someone to hold and caress.

But just being aware of how unsatisfying pictures can be was not enough. For Ben it was going to be a long, hard road to undo the distortions produced by years and years of dependence on X-rated magazines, movies, and fantasies.

Is Ben alone? Not at all. Scores and scores of boys in all our neighborhoods are learning to use pornography during the waiting period as their only sexual outlet. Meanwhile, no one talks or writes about the real problem. How does a person driven by hormones avoid developing obsessional patterns of sexual behavior?

The role of guilt in modern-day sexuality. Male sexuality also goes wrong whenever early development and the long period of expected abstinence are filled with guilt-producing condemnation. There is a healthy form of guilt we must all learn, but false, neurotic guilt, on the other hand, doesn't stop bad sexual behavior; it only makes matters worse. It's hard enough for the average boy to fight a battle with raging hormones from age twelve until age twenty-five. What is he to do with the guilt created by taboos imposed by insecure or insensitive parents who know how to condemn but who can't teach the ABCs of forgiveness?

Regrettably, there will also be a disproportionate amount of guilt in children who grow up in a religious environment. Being a Christian myself, I know just how easily guilt creeps into parenting. An anonymous Christian pastor once wrote these words:

> Years from now, when socio-historians sift through the documents describing our times, they will undoubtedly come up with elegant explanations of why men who grew up in church homes are oversexed and vulnerable to attacks of lust and obsession, and why women who grew up in those same environments emerged uptight and somewhat disinterested in sex.[5]

I know these words are not easy to swallow, but they force us to think. The writer makes a very valid point. A religious upbringing is more likely to create guilt feelings about sexuality than a nonreligious one. The process goes like this: A boy feels the excitement of his sex drive. He tries to resist masturbating because he's been told he shouldn't. However, the more he tries to resist it, the greater his inner tension grows, along with the need to seek release. The guilt seems to add its own tension, raising the level of excitement.

Finally the boy masturbates. He experiences a great release, but feelings of remorse immediately follow. This drives him down to a deep low, not unlike the experience of some drug addicts who use downers to accentuate the uppers of their drug addiction.

Soon the process starts all over again. From a deep low brought on by guilt or shame, the boy's arousal climbs to a new high created by the tension of trying to resist his sexual arousal. He masturbates, and the process starts all over again. This is the dynamic that establishes the masturbation as an obsessive/compulsive habit.

Any guilt-inducing technique, without adequate instruction about human sexual response and without a clear understanding of how to be self-forgiving, will certainly create an obsessive/compulsive type of sexuality.

Many, many fine moral and good men are haunted by feelings of lust, obsessions about sex, and compulsions to masturbate. This began with extreme feelings of guilt and shame generated during their teenage years. They feel oversexed, and perhaps they are. Their obsessions and compulsions never subside, even after years of happy and sexually satisfying marriage. Only hard, dedicated work can remove them. The challenge before us is how to teach sexual self-control without creating neurotic guilt.

There's a difference between neurotic guilt and healthy guilt. Healthy guilt makes us moral people. It forces us to pay our debts on time and not steal from one another. Healthy guilt is good and necessary. The difference lies in the issue of forgiveness; neurotic guilt doesn't want to be forgiven. It demands punishment. And if no one else is there to punish us, we do it ourselves. Much depression is the result of self-punishment. Some people can't just accept the fact that they are imperfect and make mistakes.

Of course, if you know God's forgiveness at a very deep level, it helps you stop punishing yourself. But even in light of God's mercy, neurotic guilt can get in the way. I know many Christian people who simply cannot accept God's forgiveness. They go on punishing themselves, even for the slightest of human failings.

The adrenaline connection. The final mechanism that creates a dark side to male sexuality is what I call the adrenaline connection. Whenever testosterone and adrenaline become connected, you have an explosive mixture. Sex-and-adrenaline excitement may make sexual arousal more exciting, but it also makes it more dangerous. It's the stuff of which perversions are made.

Like so many men, Harvey hardly ever thinks of anything besides sex. He goes to bed thinking about it. He wakes up thinking about it. Even the spontaneous erections triggered by a full bladder upon waking remind him of sex.

Harvey's wife feels very uncomfortable about Harvey's sexual needs, and rightly so. They've been married about five years and overall have a good sexual relationship. However, Harvey is continually searching for some novel way to have sex. When they were first married, he studied all the how-to manuals and kept pressuring his wife to try different positions. No sooner had they mastered one position than Harvey was inventing something new. He needed variety to keep his sexual excitement at a high pitch.

He put pressure on his wife to try different places around the house. Upstairs, downstairs, on the porch at night. Soon these became old hat, so he pleaded with her to spend the night in a local hotel room with him.

Then he wanted to try riskier settings. He discovered that he could get a much higher arousal if there were other people nearby. For instance, when dinner guests were over, he pleaded with her to go to the bedroom with him for a "quickie." Needless to say, Harvey's wife knew there was a problem. No matter what new and novel context Harvey invented for their lovemaking, he soon got bored and needed something newer and more novel to give him excitement.

What is Harvey's problem? I believe that Harvey is hooked on two forms of arousal. First, he needs and wants his sexual needs met. But this basic arousal isn't enough for Harvey. By whatever means, he has from his earliest years of adolescence become used to a second form of arousal—adrenaline arousal. Just as some drugs magnify the effects of others, adrenaline magnifies sexual arousal.

This kind of experience can happen quite by chance if one does something risky, novel, or taboo while being sexually aroused. The risky, novel, or taboo action causes adrenaline to rush—just ask a bungee jumper, parachutist, hang glider, or other thrill-seeking person. When it comes to sex, some men try to get this adrenaline rush as intense as possible while having a sexual high. This produces a double excitement.

The problem is, it only works for a short period of time. You get used to it, so that one particular type of thrill no longer excites you. You have to move on to something even riskier. Once you get onto this merry-go-round, it's difficult to get off. It is a never-ending process of searching for newer and more stimulating activities to go along with sex.

The use of pain, either in receiving it or inflicting it as happens in sadomasochistic sex is also a creator of an adrenaline rush. This is why pain and sex have been so closely linked throughout human history. Snuffing out a life in the act of sex is the ultimate perversion and is seen in many serial killings. It is the ultimate expression of the adrenaline/ sexual connection.

Many normal and otherwise healthy men, of course, never go to these extremes. They are not so perverse as to engage in painful or dangerous sexual acts. But they can unwittingly engage in a search for ever-increasing sexual thrills by linking sex with risky behavior. Porn, places, and positions are but a few of the ways men try to get more thrills out of sex. Unfortunately there is no final, ultimate thrill to be had by an adrenaline fix. A healthy sexuality needs to be free of these addicting tendencies.

How can a man addicted to thrill-seeking activities during sex break this habit?

First, be content with basic sex. Sex is beautiful and sufficient in itself: Stop trying to find an ever-higher thrill. Accept it at its basic level of satisfaction.

Second, stop all behaviors that create an adrenaline rush during sex. Just as alcoholics must stop drinking to break their alcoholism, the sex-adrenaline junky needs to do the same. Go cold turkey.

Third, focus on building your love relationship as the foundation to sex. Sex without love is a hollow thing, which is why so many men try to fill what is missing with adrenaline arousal. Put passion back into your marriage. Build intimacy and deep friendship. Not only will these bring a genuine new depth to your sexual experience, but you will find that they are more satisfying than anything adrenaline offers you.

Fourth, if your marriage is such that it provides no real opportunity to build a satisfying sexual relationship, seek counsel for yourself. Many men wait too long before getting help for a bad marriage or for a sexual problem. The sooner you address a problem the more successful the result will be.

THE MISUSES OF SEX

Sex has many uses, and men use sex for many reasons beyond the essential satisfaction of the sex drive. The motivations and needs met through the pleasure of sex are many and not just physical; they are psychological as well. Among the more common misuses of sex are the following:

- As a tranquilizer to relieve tension and stress.

- As an antidepressant to relieve feelings of melancholy or self-pity.

- As a means of venting anger through the uncontrolled release of sexual energy.

- To prove one's masculinity and power, or to prove one's worthiness, popularity, or irresistibility.

- To dominate one's partner by taking advantage of her sexual desires.

- To prove to one's partner that you love her, especially when you are not able to express love and tenderness in other ways.

- As sensation seeking, believing that somehow in sex is to be found all the joys of human existence.

While sex can be used to meet many needs, it has its limits. Sex is not appropriate for meeting human needs that should be fulfilled in other ways.

4

How Men Think
about Sex

Men see sex everywhere. The message of sex stares at them from every magazine rack and blares at them from every television talk show. We can't escape it. There are constant reminders in every man's world that he is riding on his hormones. It is hardly surprising that men are confused about their sexuality. Sex is in too prominent a position in our existence, and thus it dominates the average male's thinking far more than it should.

Not only do men see sex everywhere, they also see sex in everything. Low-cut dresses. Tight jeans. Friendliness, and even a smile. Men have the capability of turning almost anything into a fetish that can excite erotic feelings. One minister wrote to me and told me of how he couldn't help interpreting sounds as sexual.

> Whenever I go to a conference or a retreat where there are married couples, I can't help myself. I lie awake at night listening to the sounds in the rooms next door or upstairs. The slightest creak turns me on. I get all excited. My hands shake. My chest gets tense and I start to breathe heavily. If the sound repeats itself, I become even more convinced that whoever is in the room next door or above is having sex.

It is the sound that excites me. If I walked in on someone
in the act I would probably drop dead. It wouldn't excite me at
all. But the sounds of the night seem to have some special
sexual meaning to me. Perhaps I heard my parents making love
as a child. I don't remember.

When Do Men Start Thinking about Sex?

One of the questions I asked the men in my study was about how early
in their lives they recall having their first sexual feelings. So much recon-
struction of our memory takes place in later life that it is not possible to
be absolutely accurate about recalling early childhood feelings. But I
asked the men anyway.

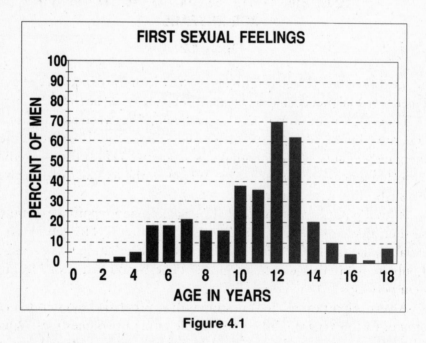

Figure 4.1

Figure 4.1 presents the results. Some men reported that their first
sexual feelings occurred as early as the age of two. This surprises me because generally we don't remember anything before age three. What these
men are saying is that it occurred right at the beginning of their memory.
The majority of men reported that their first feelings occurred between

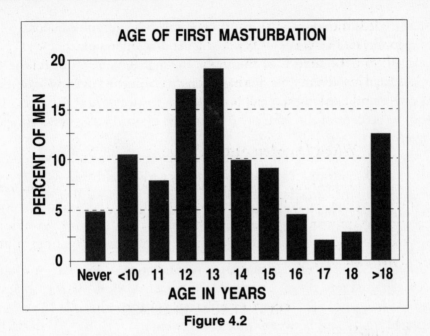

Figure 4.2

the ages of ten and thirteen. This agrees well with the experience of most of men—sexual preoccupation begins just before or at the time of puberty.

There is a slight drop in first sexual feelings between ages eight and nine, the prepuberty years. At this age, boys seem to pull away from their emerging sexuality. This may simply be a defense against the awakening to the differences between the sexes. Whatever the reason, there seems to be a slight drop at this time.

A final point is worth noting also. Several men reported experiencing their first sexual feelings as late as age eighteen. This late onset of sexual thoughts corresponds to a late start in masturbation. How does age of puberty relate to age of first feelings? Puberty and first sexual feelings occur very close to each other.

A very important related question is this: When do boys start to masturbate? In this regard, I asked my sample of men two questions: When did you first start masturbating? And, by age sixteen, how often do you estimate you masturbated *per month*.

First, let me report on how many men say they *did not* masturbate in their youth. It may seem alarming that so many masturbated, since my sample comprises mainly "good" men who have been raised in Christian homes. Yet less than 5 percent of the sample reported that they had never masturbated in their youth! In other words, 95 percent of males, even from good, healthy, religious families *admit to masturbating*.

Figure 4.2 shows the distribution of the masturbation-starting age. It ranges from age ten to over age eighteen. Some started as early as seven. As one would expect, the peak is between ages twelve and thirteen. Almost 80 percent of the men say they started masturbating between ages eleven and fifteen.

It is very clear from my data that the majority of men, 95 percent in fact, started masturbating in their youth or early adulthood. This is certainly consistent with the anecdotal findings of my clinical work. When I report this in some religious circles, however, people respond as if it were unbelievable.

How *frequently* do boys masturbate?

Figure 4.3 reports the frequency of masturbation at age sixteen. Quite a few reported zero times per month (23 percent). Most (48 percent) reported a frequency of between five and ten times a month while 13 percent reported that it was between fifteen and twenty.

How does this inform us about how men think? Clearly, boys from age twelve onward are giving a lot of attention to their urges and are constantly being reminded by their hormones that they are sexual creatures.

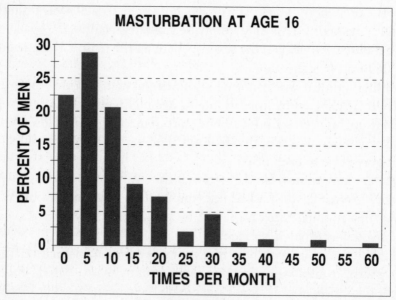

Figure 4:3

More than three out of four (77 percent) of them masturbate more than five times a month, and some as frequently as twice a day.

What do they *think* about as they masturbate? What do they look at? What fantasies are fostered? If a dependency on both fantasy and visual stimuli develops in these early years, it will be difficult to break later in life. And its impact on sexual development is a lot more serious than most people realize.

What Influences Male Sexual Thinking?

There are many influences that condition the unique way a male thinks about sex. Some understanding of these influences can help us become better parents as we try to teach our children, especially our sons and grandsons, healthier ways to be sexual. Here are three of these influences, involving repression of emotions, repression of sensuality, and being "real men."

Repression of emotions. Upon seeing an attractive girl, boys are aware, on the one hand, of their sexual arousal. But they do not learn to identify their deeper accompanying feelings. They learn to separate the two. Arousal is not a feeling, for males; it is a *sensation*: accelerated heartbeat, exhilaration, excitement. Feelings are not just sensations; they are *more* than sensations and have to do with the *meanings* we attach to sensations. Males learn very early to keep the two separated. They understand the sensations of sexual arousal but shut out the accompanying feelings.

Is this healthy? Clearly not. We are more than animals. Animals just experience sensations, not feelings. They can perform sexual acts in the open without any embarrassment whatsoever. And unless we raise our boys with greater attention to their awareness of feelings, sex will remain animalistic for them. Without the awareness of feelings such as tenderness, love, gentleness, consideration, and sympathy, sex is brutish and animalistic.

Herein lies a major difference between the sexuality of males and females. Females learn to connect their feelings with their sexuality. Males don't, especially when they grow up in an emotionally repressed environment. And when all their feelings are repressed, their sexuality becomes split off from these feelings as well.

Repression of sensuality. The sensuality of sex should be as important to men as it generally is to women. It is what makes sex healthy. Sex without sensuality merely reduces it to an act in which release is the primary objective. The male who lacks sensuality also lacks sensitivity and is unable to serve as a satisfactory sexual partner because he doesn't enjoy the broader experience of sex. If he isn't getting intercourse he isn't happy. He's never satisfied with anything less.

How does this come about? By depriving boys of the basic building blocks of sensuality—kissing, hugging, touching, stroking, being close to another. These experiences are sensual because they have to do with our senses. They do not, of themselves, constitute anything sexual. But for sexuality to be sensual, a boy, and later a man, must feel comfortable with these basic building blocks.

Every therapist who has worked with sexual dysfunction knows how important it is to recover or develop these basic building blocks in the male. Women find it easier than men because while growing up they've been loved more overtly. We hug and kiss girls more than we do boys. But boys need hugging, too. They need to be kissed by both parents. Physical contact of a nonsexual nature helps to open up sexual touching later.

A man who has been deprived of these building blocks won't approach his wife with loving thoughts about how he can create a sensual atmosphere. He will be goal-oriented, all business about his sex life, just as he is about his work. He'll probably believe that all females think the way he does, so he'll get mad if he doesn't achieve his goal.

Being "Real Men." Boys are also influenced by a strong compulsion to prove their masculinity.[1] How do they do this? Boys are taught to believe that they must prove themselves through how they perform. Their self-esteem, fragile at best, becomes totally dependent upon how well they do.

Some men can't enjoy the journey, or even the moment of sex, because they are too concerned about the destination. And if a man's performance falters, his anxiety skyrockets while his confidence takes a plunge. The male ego is so wrapped up in performance that lack of it cripples him.

How does this show up in the male's thinking about sex? For one, women are judged by their potential to facilitate his performance in success or failure. When a husband doesn't feel like he is being very successful as a lover he pulls back and avoids his wife. His thoughts either dwell on his failure or focus on blaming his wife. This has led many a male to seek out an easy-success experience—a casual acquaintance he meets on a business trip, a paid escort, someone inferior socially that he can use for his own immediate sexual goal gratification.

Anxiety over sexual performance in the male also shows itself in a tendency to believe that he must be ready for sex at all times. The success of lovemaking depends on him alone. This performance compulsion will push him to try, even when he's not ready. Why? Because in his thinking, real men are always ready. Such a man then seeks constant stimulation, such as pornography, to keep himself at peak readiness.

I have worked in therapy with several men who have developed such a habit. As they get older their sexual readiness has declined, but their male egos have not adjusted. So they spend their days eying attractive women, seeking all the sexual stimulation they can get, soaking up every drop of arousal, peeking at every bit of exposed flesh, and concocting elaborate fantasies. All this is done with the intention of raising their sexual readiness for the moment when performance is required of them. They can't just let it happen in low gear; they must keep their engine running at peak revs. As one might imagine, their preoccupation with success almost guarantees frequent failure.

How Often Do Men Think about Sex?

This is an intriguing and much-debated question. Susan Bakos says that the average man has eight sexual fantasies per hour, "ranging from his fleeting erotic appreciation of a passing pair of legs to mental images of penetration."[2] I doubt if this is universally true. From the way she writes, I wonder if she's talking about a certain type of man, not the good men I am describing here.

But good or bad, the fact is that a man thinks about sex a lot, though it varies from day to day, depending on whether he has just had sex or not, on the level of his stress at work, and on other factors. Still, the "how often?" question is an important one.

Reckoning with some variability from day to day, I asked my sample of men how often their thoughts turn to sex. All they had to do was indicate the time interval from about once a year, a month, a week, daily, hourly, or every minute. They even had the option of answering "never." In this way I hoped to find out what time period most men frequently associated

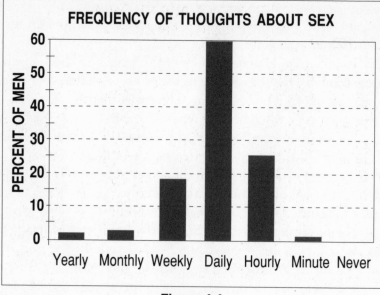

Figure 4.4

with thoughts about sex. The question is very subjective and probably has a projective element in it—but it is the best I could do.

Figure 4.4 presents the results. No one answered "never." Sooner or later all men think about sex. A not insignificant number of men (16 percent) reported that they thought about it hourly. Most (more than 61 percent in fact) answered "daily," and this agrees well with my clinical experience. Combining those men who thought about sex daily or more frequently accounts for almost 80 percent of all men. This is a lot of thought power being given to sex.

In the way I worded the question, I believe that men were answering the question with respect to their own sexuality, not abstractly or about other people's issues. It was their feelings, desires, fantasies, fleeting erotic arousals, or something they saw that turned their minds to sex. And four out of five men said that hardly a day goes by when they are not thinking about sex.

Is this normal? Absolutely, it is. There is nothing immoral about thinking of sex. Just having our minds drift toward sex is perfectly normal, given the high level of exposure we have to stimulating triggers in our culture.

What we do with these thoughts is another matter. If our thoughts feed lustful preoccupation or obsessions about a particular person, or distract us from work, then they may not be healthy. But just having our minds remind

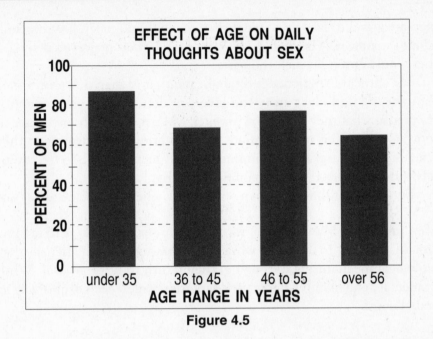

Figure 4.5

us of sex is a sign that we are alive and our endocrine systems are connected to our brains.

After analyzing the frequency with which male thinking turns to sex, I
immediately asked myself: Is the frequency in any way tied to age? In other
words, do younger men tend to think about sex more often than older men?
I have noticed a slight decline in this frequency in myself as I've gotten
older, but I wondered about others. So I analyzed the responses and came
up with the chart in Figure 4.5. As a study of this chart will show, there is a
slight trend downward with age. Not much, but noticeable. A higher percentage of men under age thirty-five seemed to have thoughts about sex
on a daily or hourly frequency (86 percent) than those over fifty-six (65
percent). This seems consistent with my experience. So, with age comes
a slight decrease in the frequency with which we think about sex.

When It Comes to Sex, What Do Men Think About?

This is a more difficult question to answer. First of all, men differ
widely in the content of their sexual thoughts. Secondly, they don't like
revealing the real content of their innermost secrets. In fact most good

men are afraid to face up to what they really think, much less to openly admit it. Some may be shocked by what I say. Others may even deny that they would entertain such thoughts.

My clinical experience has taught me that as men delve into their thought life and clear away the layers of denial, they are frequently alarmed at what they discover. However, when men with honesty face up to what is going on in their minds, it often brings deep healing to their sexuality. Guilt and shame diminish so that men are able to free themselves from the obsessions or compulsions that haunt them.

But what is it that good men really think when they think about sex?

Men fantasize. Men fantasize for many reasons. They do it to achieve arousal, learning to do it first while masturbating as boys. Then, as their biological mechanisms start aging, they return to it for arousal. While women depend mainly on romantic fantasies, males reach exclusively for sexual ones.

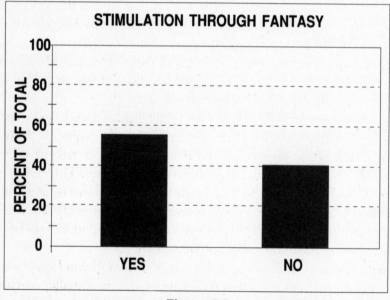

Figure 4.6

To what extent do men fantasize about having sex with someone other than their partner in order to achieve stimulation? This is always a sore point for wives. I put this question to my male sample, and Figure 4.6 is the result. While not overwhelming, 57 percent of these men admitted to achieving stimulation through fantasy of another person. Most of the rest (41 percent) said they didn't. Curiously, quite a few refused to answer the question. I suppose I really should count these in with those who do, because if they don't, why wouldn't they say so?

Men who fantasize about having sex with other women don't necessarily see it as cheating or swapping. They are just intrigued by the fantasy. Some even say it helps them to remain faithful. One patient told me once, "It helps for me to fantasize having sex with others. That way I satisfy my interests in other women and don't have to be unfaithful!"

Since he was a deeply religious man, I reminded him that even if adultery is committed in the mind, it is still sinful. His response? "I don't want to talk about it."

Dependence on fantasy for sexual arousal is extremely common in men. It may not always involve having sex with someone else. It doesn't always indulge sizzling sexual encounters. Sometimes it's just imagining that you are in a special place with your partner or doing a special thing. I have no problems with such fantasies. They may genuinely enrich a relationship.

But there are fantasies and there are fantasies. When they involve your appropriate partner, they may be good. But if they take liberties with others they are of doubtful value. The *excessive* use of fantasy seems to me to be an unhealthy thing for several reasons.

First, fantasy is not reality. I think that the repeated escape into a fantasy world avoids closeness with your partner in the here and now. It avoids intimacy: the full experience of your true self with your true partner.

Second, fantasy is addictive. All addictions habituate. This means that you get so used to the substance or behavior that you have to increase the dose or frequency for it to give you pleasure. Fantasy is an addiction that just keeps growing and growing. The more you use it, the more you have to have it, and the further it takes you from reality.

Third, fantasy often leads to acting out. Let me tell you Bernie's story. Bernie had a good marriage. He and his wife were quite sexually compatible. But Bernie took little time to develop an intimate relationship with his wife. No romantic dinners. No long strolls through the park. No deep, personal conversations. Never time for a date or an outing alone. So their sex became just a ritual of release—every three or four days Bernie did his thing.

Since there were no romantic preliminaries leading to arousal, Bernie began fantasizing about prostitutes. He imagined driving along a lonely road and seeing a girl in a short dress. She's there just for him. She smiles and beckons. Bernie stops and picks her up. And so on. I really don't need to spell out all the details, do I?

Bernie's imagination, however, has its limits in bringing satisfaction. One day he begins to think, "I wonder what it would be like to actually go to bed with someone like that? Surely there are other men who do this. Respectable men." Slowly his fantasies became more than fantasies. They became longings—yearnings.

Bernie began to obsess about going to bed with a prostitute. On his way home from work he would drive through a neighborhood where he had heard prostitutes hang out. He was shocked to see that they were real unsavory characters. The girls in his dreams were always respectable despite their occupation. He felt ashamed. How could he be attracted to these sluts? He went back to his fantasy world—for a time.

Then one day on a business trip Bernie was approached in the hotel lobby by quite a presentable lady. Attractive, friendly, and she seemed to like him. She just walked up and said, "Hi!" Was he free that night? Did he want a good time? He was blinded by her seductive approach. This was his fantasy come true. Before he realized it she was with him in his hotel room—obviously a call girl on the make. Then the fantasy bubble burst. She wanted to know how much he was going to pay her. Money? He'd never ever paid his fantasy girls!

Fortunately Bernie came to his senses before things went too far. Revolted at what he was doing, he gave her some money and excused her by saying he was feeling sick. He was. After she had left he threw up in the bathroom.

The experience cured Bernie of his dependence on fantasies. They may seem innocent enough at first, but when you become too dependent on them, they aren't much different than any other drug.

Another thought—fantasies involve other people with whom you are taking liberties. You don't have their permission to include them in your mental sex. There is something indecent, then, in using them for your pleasure. The only way we, as men, will ever get over always seeing women as sexual objects is to stop using them to satisfy our sexual fantasies. Fantasy is not as innocent as some would make it out to be. In many subtle ways it shapes our sexual attitudes and creates appetites that are best left dormant.

Men think visually. Someone has said that whereas women are possessed by the chemistry that drives their bodies, men are driven by their hormones. There's a lot of truth here. What it means is that whereas a woman's body is possessed by a *complex* array of chemical activities that not only control the sexual response but the reproductive response also, *men only have one system*, their sexual hormones, controlling them.

Female sexuality, at least from a biological and chemical point of view, is much more complex than male sexuality. But it is also complex from a psychological point of view. Nowhere is the difference between the sexes more obvious than in the way men use vision as a sexual aid.

Men are visual. Men are attracted to what they see. They are drawn to pictures, especially of nudity. Men are attracted to pornography partly because it satisfies this visual need. I'm not saying that this attraction is normal, just that it's common.

Before the advent of the VCR, sexually oriented video material was some-what limited for most men to ordinary movies that depicted nudity or sexual activities. Now this has changed and hard-core porn is finding its way into nearly all homes. The trend to bring this type of stimuli into the home has not escaped good men. Even pastors have been attracted to this readily available source of stimulation. And it is affecting how they think and behave.

This readily available visual stimulation is increasing the male's dependence on visual stimuli, which is already very strong. Now it is becoming necessary for sexual arousal itself. What's wrong with this? It means male sexual thoughts are focused on pictures, moving or still, not on the experience of one's real relationship. In this sense, it is an intrusion into the union of the partners.

Yes, the male's thoughts are strongly dependent on visual stimuli. But where should this stimulation come from, his wife or some other image? To stay within the bounds of normality and do justice to the partner we profess to love, we must draw the line somewhere.

This brings me to yet another concern I have about the male's thought-life. Just around the corner, about to be perfected and made available on a large scale, is the wonderfully new experience of "virtual reality." Wonderful? It depends on what you use it for.

Virtual here means "as good as the real thing." *Virtual reality* is the computer's way of simulating the sights, sounds, and feelings of imaginary worlds. It is all possible through the magic of powerful minicomputers.

Virtual reality will have many wonderful benefits. It will be a fantastic teaching tool. Kids can go back in time and travel with Marco Polo or move into the future and go to the moon. Whether we're planning vacations, studying, or recreating, we'll never be the same again once virtual reality is available to all of us.

How will virtual reality affect men's thinking about sexuality? Believe me, the pornography industry will jump on this opportunity. Choose your sexual partner from the variety shown on your computer screen and settle down for an evening of fun! It will all be so close to reality that your brain won't know the difference.

Is this just science fiction? Not at all. The May 31, 1993, issue of *Newsweek* says it's just around the corner. We are well on the way to this next phase in our sexual experience. And you can be sure of this—it will drive men and women even further apart.

Men think dirty. As I have worked with highly moral and genuinely good men, I have been struck again and again by the fact that men's mental sexual soundtrack never matches the high moral tone of their behavior. This soundtrack is seldom heard outside the intimacy of the therapist's office. If it were, it certainly wouldn't bring an encouraging word to their wives.

Sexual thoughts are often free-floating. As long as a man doesn't dwell on these thoughts, he remains a healthy and highly moral man. I need to stress this point because so many good men are bothered by the intrusiveness and obscenity of their unchosen sexual thoughts. These thoughts are extinguished more by ignoring them than by giving them attention.

We are not directly responsible for the intrusion of unsavory thoughts into our thinking. It is our responsibility, however, to displace these unsavory thoughts by dwelling on cleaner ones. This is the import of those beautiful verses from Philippians 4:8–9:

> Whatever is true, whatever is noble, whatever is right, whatever
> is pure, whatever is lovely, whatever is admirable—if anything
> is excellent or praiseworthy—think about such things. (NIV)

A very close friend once shared with me a very real, very common concern. Let's call him Murray. Murray is a deeply committed Christian believer. Converted after graduating from high school, he went into the trucking business and soon owned his own company. He worked hard and was rewarded with great success. He has a well-balanced life, a lovely wife, and good kids. So what's his problem?

Murray is bothered by the way he thinks. Obscene, sexual thoughts haunt him. It all started after he was converted and began going to church. He was in the sanctuary enjoying the beauty of the service when suddenly a visual image of a nude female flashed on the screen of his mind. He was flabbergasted. Sure, he was a normal young man with strong sexual urges. He'd fooled around a bit in high school—heavy petting, no more. Never had he seen such a vivid sexual image.

Murray tried to push the image out of his mind. Actually, he was more repulsed than aroused. A few minutes later, it was back again. The more he tried to erase the thought from his mind, the more vividly it would recur.

For a few weeks following this first episode, although he was afraid to go to church, nothing happened. Then, one day the image was back again. "I must not think sexual thoughts in church," he said to himself over and over again. The more he lectured himself, the stronger the images became. Eventually, Murray could not sit in a church without these sexual images and thoughts jumping into his mind.

Years later, happily married, he was still struggling with the same dilemma. He wondered if perhaps it was a spiritual problem. "Perhaps I'm possessed," he tentatively suggested in one of our conversations. "Maybe I'm a lecherous man because something evil possesses me."

"Not likely," I told him. There was a more natural explanation. I told him the story of the man who said to a friend, "Whatever you do, don't think about a white bear." The poor man was then driven to distraction because he couldn't stop thinking about a white bear. The harder he tried the more difficult it was to get the white bear out of his mind. Try the experiment yourself.

The parallel here is obvious. When, out of a high sense of morality, you say to yourself, "Don't think about sex when you're on holy ground," you're bound to have intrusive thoughts about sex. That's how the human mind works. How can you cure this problem? Just ignore the intrusive thoughts. Don't reinforce them by being concerned. God knows what is going on. Thoughts just happen, and they are not a reflection of who we really are unless we make them so.

As I have already explained, sex is never far away in a healthy male's mental experience. Testosterone sees to this. When a man is sexually aroused, he doesn't like to talk about love so much. He prefers to think about the graphic pictures in his mind. Men think such thoughts to keep the flames burning. The more graphic the thoughts, the hotter the fire.

There is a tendency, then, in the intimate moments of sexuality for a man to become coarse and crude. And this isn't only true for blue-collar workers whose conversations are more likely to be sprinkled with frank language anyway. Even the courteous professional may drop the facade of respectability and resort to frank, even crude, thoughts and language in moments of passion.

Some wives become upset by this. One wife told me that she thought her husband had two personalities. No, what he has is a public and a very private world that he keeps far apart. In passion, the thoughts of his private world break through his defenses.

In a similar vein, a lot of the thinking that goes on behind the outwardly pleasant male conversation, tête-á-tête, and jovial storytelling is about sex. If his private thoughts were broadcast over a P.A. system as they occurred, they would sound like this: "I wonder how she is in bed?" "When did she last have sex?" "I wonder if she wants me?" Men sexually objectify women in their thoughts, while women tend to romanticize men.

Men see women as a collection of body parts, not as people. The feminist movement is right when it complains about how men view women. But no amount of fussing about this is going to change it—only a dramatic change in the way the male brain is programmed will effect any change. In the meantime, we can demand right behavior while we reprogram ourselves along the lines I am discussing in this book.

Men enjoy dirty humor. The dirty patterns of male thinking show up most clearly in the area of sexual humor. Because vulgar sexual humor is so very common in male circles, it deserves some comment here.

Watch any TV comedy channel and you will find that 50 percent of the comedians get their laughs merely by making crude comments about sexual anatomy or the acts of sex. Sadly, comediennes are now doing the same. There needn't be a story, or even a punch line. Just say something obscene and people laugh.

Male humor is direct, bawdy, and unashamed. It gets laughs because it reflects the direct opposite of male behavior. In other words, it reveals the private thoughts of the male, not his actions. It makes explicit what men think but never say, and it comes across as immature and juvenile, which is what it is. The sexual thought-life of the average male is often rude and crude, fixated in early adolescence.

Now I'm not a prude. I've laughed at my share of sexual jokes. But I have always felt uneasy doing so because of a sneaking suspicion that something deeper was going on. Think about some of the jokes you have laughed at. Don't they tell you something about yourself?

It's no puritanical preoccupation that raises my concerns about male sexual thinking, especially about male humor. It is being a grandfather to three beautiful boys and three gorgeous girls and wondering how healthy they are going to be when they grow up if we don't do something to change our world.

I've tried to come to terms with and resolve most of my own sexual distortions and hang-ups. I only wish I could protect my grandchildren from experiencing their twisted world the way that most of us did. Male sexuality deserves better treatment than we give it. It doesn't have to mutilate or disfigure the male ego. And yes, you can be healthy without becoming a nerdish prude—it's hard, but it's possible. We know what needs to be done. All we need is the courage to do it.

HOW MALES DIFFER FROM FEMALES IN THEIR SEXUALITY

Men and women seem doomed to speak different sexual languages. Men, on the one hand, speak and hear a language of confrontation and independence. They show little emotion and stick to few words, like "yup" and "nope." When they do speak they are externally oriented and focused. Men think "fix it, solve it, do it."

Women speak in softer tones with more affection and verbal approval. The differences come from the way we are raised. Girls whisper secrets while boys run, hit, and grab. This pretty well sums up their different approaches to sex as well. Here are some of the major differences between the sexes:

1. Women like to touch; men like to feel.

2. Women enjoy being courted; men prefer to get going.

3. Women like to talk about their love; men prefer to show it by action.

4. Women like the ambiance to be right: subdued light, candles, soft music, and flowers. Men prefer bright lights, loud music, and even having the TV on during sex.

5. Women like to take their time, savoring each moment, each touch. Men are "get it over quickly" compulsives.

6. Men like morning sex. They're rested and wake up with an erection. Women prefer a late-evening rendezvous with time for preparation.

7. Men want sex more frequently than women. Quantity is preferred over quality for men.

8. Men are adventurous; they like to explore and experiment. Women find one way that is most comfortable and prefer to stick with it.

9. Men take sexual rejection very personally, no matter how gently it is presented. Their masculinity is integral to their sexuality.

10. On one point men and women don't differ: they both derive tremendous excitement from seeing their partners being satisfied.

5

What Men Really Want from Sex

I t is a very common belief that what separates men and women is what each wants out of sex. I say "belief" because I'm not convinced that their desires are so different. It's as if both sexes are traveling to a distant city. They both know where they want to go; they just choose different means for getting there.

I can't really answer the "What do you really want?" question for women. I know what my wife wants. I know what several of my female clients want. But in general, I'm no expert about female sexuality. However, I do have an inkling of what it is that men want.

A recent article in *Newsweek* by Sandra Crichton, along with other staff writers, accurately describes the current confusion that exists between sexes about what each really wants.

> Behind all the hype about what is appropriate behavior in the workplace, on college campuses, or even in married couples' bedrooms, is the more basic question: What do men really want from sex? Rape and sexual harassment are real and disgraceful. But criminalizing sexuality by over-specifying what can or cannot be done only confuses the behavior of sexuality further. Between sexual bliss and crime are some cloudy waters that only re-education may help to clear.[1]

Let's be honest. Sex is inherently dangerous, and nature has given the deadliest weapon to men. Hazards lie not only in the pain of forced sex but in the "exposure to everything from euphoria to crashing disappointment."[2] There is great unpredictability in sex.

It is the male who has traditionally initiated sex, and even in our modern world often still does. And according to everything I have observed and studied, it is the male who desperately needs to understand himself and be understood by others in these revolutionary times. Only out of this understanding can come a new agenda for raising males to behave in a civilized way when it comes to sex.

The Battle with Sexuality

Not all boys turn out to be Tailhook-style grabbers, points-gathering football jocks, or sex-crazed chauvinists. But they all come to maturity with a lot of distortion surrounding their sexuality. To guarantee the propagation of the human race, the laws of nature are programmed to enforce procreation by a mighty irresistible urge toward sensuality. Or, to put it bluntly, men love to have sex! They are designed for it. Like it or not, if you are a male, chances are you've inherited an impulse so strong and a desire so overbearing at times that you sometimes think you're going crazy. Is this normal? I can guarantee that it is, up to a point.

Sure, we'd like to believe that sexuality has higher motives and aims. We don't want to see ourselves on the same level as beasts who just seek to gratify primitive lust or instinct. We want to believe that there are higher motives in sex, such as building intimacy and tenderness, generating offspring who can build a better world, and enhancing marital bliss. But the truth is that the sex drive and its powerful hormones dominate and even distort the action we would like to see take place.

Most men face a lifelong struggle to control their sexuality. The struggle is between their hormones and their higher aspirations. It is a battle between their seemingly uncontrollable urges and the fear of succumbing to these urges. Ultimately, it is a struggle over integrity, right and wrong, uprightness, and wholeness. To put it in a simple word, it is a struggle to be "good."

I have no patience with those who berate the pastor, rabbi, or priest for falling into sexual sin. Those who are quick to throw stones need to

look at themselves. Furthermore, to suggest that it is because of their religious leanings that they have set themselves up for sexual promiscuity
reveals an ignorance of the facts. Critics point to TV evangelists and say,
"You see, all religious zealots are sexual perverts. It's religion that does it."
Meanwhile, they turn a blind eye to the hordes of nonreligious men who
cheat on their wives, abandon families for younger partners, or just sleep
around. It's a double standard. If you're nonreligious you can do what you
like. If you're religious you must not be human.

I have worked in therapy with many pastors who have succumbed to
sexual temptations. With *very few exceptions*, they have been good men,
men I would trust with my life. They have lost the battle because the odds
were stacked against them. The miracle, in my opinion, is that so few fall.

One pastor described the battle this way to me: "How can I be a man
of the cloth and be so driven by an unbridled sex drive?" For some, it is
even a battle for sanity. "My sexual desires are driving me crazy," is how a
prominent businessman described it to me. "I sometimes wish I'd get pros-
tate cancer just so I'd have an excuse to get castrated." Of course, he was
wrong about the castration. Prostatectomy hardly ever involves that radical a surgery. But his desperation is evident.

How should men deal with their guilt feelings over their sexuality? By
all means, *feel* guilty if you do something that violates your moral standards.
I call this "true guilt." Cry, repent, make amends. Such guilt is healthy.
But don't, for heaven's sake, go on punishing yourself. Take forgiveness
and let it go. More importantly, don't feel guilty about your basic sexuality. Guilt-based sexual feelings are ingrained at an early age by unwitting
parents. One must learn to ignore these feelings.

The Distortion of Male Sexual Needs

When it comes to human sexuality, the various messages that are sent
to kids are cloaked in myth and fantasy. Some parents don't do a good job
of raising boys to be responsible for the way they express their sexuality.
They may even bring up their boys to believe it's cool to "score."

Young men get tremendous status from the aggressive pursuit of a female. I recall one father who became quite upset when he discovered his
seventeen-year-old son was still a virgin. "What?" he roared. "You're

seventeen and you're a failure already!" This father believed that it was every boy's responsibility to deflower some innocent girl before he could claim to be a man. Of course, he was not of the religious ilk like myself, but he isn't unusual. Intercourse was this macho father's idea of the male initiation rite. In front of me, during a family therapy session, he even offered to get a "high-class prostitute" to do the job for his son! Fortunately, the son had more sense and maturity than his father, so he declined the offer.

Other boys have an opposite problem. Their parents either try to indoctrinate them with fear or they refuse to discuss the topic of sex at all, leaving their sons to learn what they can from their peers. Such boys have lots of shame-based sexual feelings.

Both extremes are unhealthy, and both are common. Is it any wonder, then, that men really don't know what they want from sex? No one has taught them what to expect, and frequently they find themselves using sex to meet unhealthy needs. Here are a few ways that can happen.

Some men use sex to prove their masculinity. Men feel tremendous pressure to prove that they are adequate as men. They do this through succeeding in business and sports and through talking tough and boasting. They also do it through sex—especially through sex. Sex has long been a major arena in which to assert one's manhood. Zilbergeld warns that this often forces a man to try functioning in an unfavorable situation, thus violating the conditions for good sex. "They try to have more sex than their hormones can support, pushing themselves too much. The result is always disastrous. Sooner or later their organs stop functioning."[3]

Some men, caught in an unhappy or sexually unsatisfying marriage, may initiate an extramarital affair to prove their masculinity. They may not be able to perform in their marriage, so they assure themselves that everything is working by having an affair. Of course, trying to perform with a stranger with guilt hanging over their head and the fear of discovery doesn't create the most favorable conditions for sex. Many men come out of such an experience with even greater doubts about their masculinity. It is wiser to face up to marital unhappiness and get help than to use sex for proving anything.

Men also equate sexual frequency with masculinity. They imagine that other men are more active than they, and they may have gathered their information from that great source of all wisdom on sexual matters, the movies. Film stars always seem to be ready, willing, and able. Consequently, ordinary males find themselves wondering if something is missing or whether they are real men. They push themselves to have more sex, which may even lead to the domination of a partner. This is hardly conducive to building a satisfactory sexual relationship with a spouse.

Some men use sex as a substitute for love. Unfortunately, many men find that sex is the only way they can express love. It's the only love language they know. They have enough problems with feelings and how to express them anyway, so how can they possibly make an exception with love? It is quite common for this kind of a man to be attentive and communicative with his partner before and during sex, and to fall silent afterward. This is a major cause of wives' marital unhappiness. A woman yearns for communication, love, and attention at times other than when she is being seduced.

There are several points I want to make here. As we've noted before, there is nothing unusual about men feeling that they can have sex without the love component. I have had some married men tell me that they don't love their wives anymore but still have good sex with them. This, regrettably, is how men are programmed. Women are different.

This leads me to my second point. Whenever we talk about love we get into confusing waters. We use the phrase too loosely. We have one word for the same human feeling that we experience toward a child, a friend, a lover, and ice cream. We love them all. But we don't feel the same about all of them. Each is different—but our language only has one label for it.

What then, is love in marriage? It starts out as romantic, passionate love, heavy on the sexual juices. But this early love is just a temporary form of insanity. It attracts male to female and gets the whole dating business going. What's wrong with this? One cannot expect to remain romantically in love for the next fifty years. What is supposed to happen, though few newlyweds are told this, is that this infatuation or romantic love has to change. It must mature, grow up, become less erotic and more friendship-based. Passion must be used to build intimacy, and both must be cemented with commitment. Otherwise, love dies.

We call this process the "maturing" of love. When love matures, marital love is a very special type of friendship and closeness. Regrettably, these days, not a lot of couples persist in marriage long enough to get to this stage. It takes a long time. Along the way, you get a lot of sharp corners knocked off your raspy personality, you loosen your uptightness, and you learn to calm your bad moods. Finally, if you hang on, you discover deep, abiding love. And good sex depends, ultimately, on getting to this level of love in a relationship.

There's nothing dull about this love. It is profoundly romantic. It knows how to touch, to feel. Its sensuality is all-embracing. It can find as much pleasure in a hug or holding hands as in intercourse. This is the kind of love that knows no substitute. Sadly, few find it.

Meanwhile, women are often heard to say, "I wish he would just once in a while show me he cares without it leading to sex." They are confused by a man's sexuality. Why does every touch have to have a sexual connotation? Why must every verbal expression of love have to be seductive? The sexual relationship, and ultimately the full experience of sexual pleasure, is less than satisfactory when the male cannot find it in himself to be loving without turning it into sex.

There's a further aspect to this. As Zilbergeld points out, sometimes a man thinks that sex is a good way of finding out how a woman loves him.[4] This proof of love occurs when a man tries to get his wife—and often this technique is used coercively in dating—to show how much she cares by performing in a particular way for him. "If you really loved me, then you'd . . ." If the woman doesn't cooperate, he assumes it means she doesn't love him. Manipulative! Yet a man plays this game again and again to test how much he is loved. Of course a wise woman will turn this around and say, "If *you* really loved me, *you* wouldn't ask me to do something I don't want to do."

Sadly, some women feel coerced into cooperation because they fear losing a man's love. The fact is, no man has a right to use sex as a substitute for love or to demand it as proof of love. He should learn to express love in nonsexual ways. He will then discover that there is more to a relationship with a woman than just the act of sex—something ever so much more meaningful.

Some men use sex to satisfy addictive needs. While I don't intend to address the topic of full-blown sexual addictions in this book, clearly sex can take on all the characteristics of an addiction. All addictions have one thing in common: they function as an emotional anesthesia. They serve to kill the pain of unpleasant emotions or experiences. People resort to addictions to numb their pain or to escape from life's responsibilities. This is true for substance addictions such as alcohol or cocaine as well as for hidden addictions like gambling, shopping, or excessive TV watching. The addict uses the behavior as a form of escape from life's realities.

Because sex provides tremendous pleasure, it easily becomes a means of escape. It is both a tranquilizer for anxiety and a stimulant to provide a boost during a depressed mood. Either way, it provides an escape from some of life's more painful realities. And some men turn to sex to relieve their tension and stress.

Meaningful stress actually serves to sublimate the sex drive. But there's another form of stress that doesn't provide any meaningful involvement—the stress of worry and anxiety. It is the stress of being hassled, of having a boss on your back, of failing projects, or of difficult coworkers. This type of stress doesn't sublimate the sex drive; it makes it more intense. Sex becomes the only good thing left in life. It becomes a pacifier, a security blanket, a nirvana. And if men can't get it at home, they'll look for it somewhere else.

I was reflecting recently on the number of cases I have seen over the years regarding men who have gone through a major midlife crisis. These men have thrown away beautiful families, patient and loving wives, and even major careers and taken up with younger women. I was struck by a very consistent finding: nearly all these men were in some sort of trouble in their work life. Either a business was failing, a church was not growing as they wanted it to, they were losing their competitive edge, or some other major catastrophe had occurred. In every case, there was a preceding period of intense, negative stress. Stereotypically, the other woman is younger and more sexually active than the wife, providing more intense stimulation.

And I don't recall a single case of a man in such a midlife crisis ever saying to me: "You know, doctor, I decided to leave my wife and take up with this other woman because my wife was oversexed and always wanting me to perform. My new partner doesn't care about sex. In fact, she'd rather not have it. So now I am really content." Doesn't work like this!

Troubled men seek out more sex, different sex, varieties of sex, anything that will take away the pain of failure or disillusionment. Sex is a powerful force in the human body, but it is also a powerful force in the human mind. It can be a substitute for just about anything. And men will go to almost any length to get something out of sex that it wasn't meant to provide, namely an escape from reality. When this happens, sex becomes an addiction.

In the long run then addictive sexuality never lives up to its promises. No matter how exciting it may be, you still have to come back to earth and deal with taxes, freeways, bosses from hell, and old age. Unless sex is relegated to its proper place in human experience and used for healthy reasons, it will always end up being a disappointment. Men need to know this.

What Do Men Really Want?

So much for the wrong motives. These are only a few, and there are more, to be sure; but let's turn to men's positive needs. What do men really, rightfully want from sex? Which of their needs are genuine and need to be seriously considered?

Men want a more complete sexual experience. One of the anonymous six hundred-plus questionnaires I received back had all sorts of helpful thoughts scribbled on the sides, around the top, and on the back. Thoughtful thoughts. I pulled it out from the rest of the pile because it reflected a great deal of sensitive insight into the genuine needs of the sexual male. Among other things, the respondent wrote this:

> It seems clear to me that much of our male desire for sexuality is a misplaced desire for intimacy, having gotten the two confused in our culture in puberty.

He then goes on further to suggest that it is for this reason that so many men feel unsatisfied with their sexual experience. They can never get what they really need solely through the sexual act. They have to work at developing a more complete intimacy because if they don't, they will never be deeply satisfied with sex.

Believe it or not, men want to be joined in close, intimate companionship with their partners. This recalls the ancient Greek myth that describes the real nature of love. Originally, according to this mythical story, the earth was populated by beings who were half-man, half-woman.

Swollen with pride, they rebelled against the gods. The irate Zeus split each of them in half and scattered the halves over the earth. Ever since, each half has been searching the earth for the other half, yearning for the completion we call love.

We seek a partner from the opposite sex as if to restore our completeness. Sexual attraction is the force that drives this attraction aimed at restoring our wholeness. We have deep sexual desires that may seem to be genitally based but, in fact, are emotional. Our sexual desires—emotion *and* impulse—are functions of the highest level of our beings.[5]

In animals it may be pure instinct. In humans it is some instinct, but a lot of yearning, loving, needing, closeness, union, unconditional acceptance, and total abandonment. It invokes the most intimate parts of the whole body and mind. And here is the problem. So few men ever really get in touch with these deeper reaches of their sexual desire. Yet it is still what they need, even if they don't recognize it!

How does this translate to practical, everyday living?

- **Men want more than sex.** It is a mistake to assume that men just want raw sex. At a superficial level it may seem that this is all they want, but don't be put off by this superficial desire. They yearn for more than the basic appeasement of their testosterone. In some wonderful way their brains are programmed to seek out a more complete experience, a deep union of souls, and total harmony with another.

- **Men don't always know what they want or how to get it.** It is a mistake to assume that men know how to find what they really want, or even to assume that they know what it is. They need and want to discover the source of their deepest cravings. This journey of discovery takes time and patience. It needs an understanding environment. It takes lots of listening, not judging. It thrives in an atmosphere of acceptance, not rejection.

- **Men confuse emotional needs with sexual needs.** Every male comes into adulthood, like the female, with a host of unmet needs from childhood. Needs for unconditional love. Needs that determine self-acceptance and self-esteem.

Sexual needs often get confused with these unfulfilled needs. Men need help in sorting out the unmet emotional needs from urgent sexual needs.

- **Men have difficulty opening their hearts and baring their souls.** The tendency of males to close up emotionally is primarily the consequence of early-childhood modeling. As far as possible, men need to undo this early damage before it destroys their present lives. It takes a good listener to help a man do this. One man I know, and to some extent it was my own experience as well, learned very early to squash his feelings and never to mention them. He still hears his father's voice saying, "You sound like a sissy girl. You're just like your mother, squealing all the time. Try behaving like a man!"

- **Men long to open up emotionally.** Men really want to be open about their deep, inner selves. They want to bare it all. They just don't know how to do it. So when a male finally begins to open up it must be in the context of total acceptance with no condemnation. Men strike me as being more fragile at a deep level than women. I think this is because they don't have as much experience at handling rejection. Their inner defenses are more rigid than a woman's, but this makes them more fragile. They may appear outwardly to be tougher, but that's only because they know how to deflect deep hurts before they penetrate. Once the hurt gets in, men seem to suffer more than women.

Men want the full experience of their sexuality to be respected. Most men understand political correctness and the critical need for women to be protected from harassment and sexual crimes. But they want some understanding too.

Just as men are becoming self-conscious about their sexuality, women are becoming distrustful of all men. There is a polarization developing between the sexes. The men I have studied want a greater understanding and acceptance of their basic sexual makeup. They are not the sickies in our society. They are not the sexual addicts. They are the normal males that make up the mainstream of our society.

Men can't understand, for instance, how women can demand treatment as nonsexual objects in the workplace while dressing in a manner that is sexually provocative. "Don't they get it?" one angry pastor shouted at me once. "I have a choir director who wears the skimpiest of clothes in the summer and then complains because some of the men stare at her legs." Men can't understand why women can't understand that men are not made of ice.

One of the questions I asked a subset of my male sample (about 150 men) was, "Do you feel that women understand a man's sex drive?" Most of the men (83 percent) answered no. This no answer often reflects frustration at not getting enough sex. Most married men I know complain that their wives are not as responsive sexually as they would like them to be.

What do these good men want their partners to understand about their sexuality? Here are some of the most common messages I've been asked by frustrated husbands to communicate to their wives.

- **"I'm not abnormal."** Sometimes wives make their husbands feel like they are absolutely the most perverse, sex-crazed animals that ever walked God's earth. I know men who literally think they're going crazy because the message they receive is one of "if you were normal you wouldn't bother me as much as you do." Every couple needs to work out a satisfactory sexual schedule. I don't mean a rigid timetable; I mean a deep understanding of each other's cycle and needs. No marriage can survive and be a happy one unless there is resolution on this important issue.

- **"I can't help it if I come on strong sexually."** Many men crave a greater understanding and acceptance of the biological basis for their sex drive. They could probably control themselves better in the context of understanding than in being made to feel rejected or humiliated. "It's not my fault I was created this way," one husband pleaded with me. "Why am I always made to feel guilty?"

- **"If I inadvertently look at another woman, it doesn't mean I desire her over you."** I don't encourage men to reinforce their wandering eyes. I think men can control where they look, if only because it's good manners. Whether you're in the presence of your partner or not, self-control begins by watching your eyes!

But when a husband inadvertently glances at someone attractive, it doesn't mean the end of love has come. It just means he's alive and alert. I've known a few marriages where accidental glances like this became cause for divorce. Jealous and insecure spouses can be supervigilant and over-reactive. The problem is probably insecurity, not infidelity, so get it fixed before your marriage disintegrates.

- *"Once in a while I would like you to initiate lovemaking."* Most every man has a fantasy that involves his partner not being able to keep her hands off him—wanting him so badly that the poor woman has lost control. Very few wives, however, are geared to behave this way. There's also some doubt about how often the average man could take this sort of pressure.

  But why is this fantasy so common? I think it's because always having to initiate sex takes away some of the ex-citement. Also, men fear rejection. So in this fantasy the male just goes along for the ride. No pressure. No need to win. No risk of rejection. Just enjoyment.

  Men do get tired of doing all the courting. It's nice to know that you are desired, not doing all the desiring. Helps to make you feel normal.

- *"I like a bit of novelty now and then, and I wish you un-derstood that."* Some freshness through change is helpful, if not necessary, to every marriage. Of course the pursuit of too much novelty can be a problem if it is just for novelty's sake. Sex isn't supposed to be Fourth of July fireworks every time. Still, men would appreciate a woman's understanding about the need for variety.

- *"I don't want our kids to spoil our sexual life."* Many hus-bands feel that during the childraising stage of a marriage, sex is put on hold. This happens because of fatigue and sometimes because of worries that the kids will barge in at an inappropriate time. Just the problem of finding time for each other before you collapse out of exhaustion on the bed is a major problem. This calls for a lot of creativity, and husbands long for their wives to participate in finding creative solutions. Finding intimate moments when the kids are at a birthday party, taking them to Grandma's for the night, or getting a baby-sitter and having a date at a local motel can help to maintain sexual closeness through these trying times.

- **"Sometimes it's not sex I'm wanting, just time together."** Husbands fear that their wives are avoiding intimacy because they assume it will lead to sex. So they say "Don't touch me when I'm in the kitchen" or "Can't you see the kids in the next room?" What they really mean is "I'm not interested in sex, so keep your distance."

  I truly believe that sometimes, not always but sometimes, these men just want some physical reassurance, the comfort of giving or receiving a caress.

  Of course, men do not always just leave it there. But even when that's all they want they feel rebuffed by the cold shoulder. Touches, kisses, and caresses are needed by men also, not just women. Good sex takes a lot of nonsex time together to make it good, and men crave this more than a lot of women realize.

- **"I like to talk about our sex. Why don't you?"** I've heard women say this about their men too. But more frequently, men want to talk about their sexual responsiveness, especially in the heat of passion.

Part of the intimacy of sex is to help encourage communication during sex. Couples who say nothing miss a wonderful opportunity to free up their general communication.

"My husband never tells me he loves me. I know he does, but he never says it. I wish he would just tell me occasionally," one wife complained during a conjoint marital therapy session.

"Do you love your wife?" I asked him. "Of course I do. Very much," he replied.

"Why don't you ever tell her?" I asked.

"Often I want to," he replied, "especially when we're making love. But my wife doesn't want to talk during sex. So I've learned to keep quiet too."

"So why can't he tell me he loves me at other times?"

This was a very forthright and justified question. "If your husband can get over his shyness about love-talk during sex," I told her, "you'll eventually teach him how to love-talk you at other times." I gently tried to explain to both of them that they were missing a wonderful opportunity.

So what do men want? Understanding. Intimacy. Physical pleasure blessed with deeper meaning. It bears repeating: What men and women want from sex may not be as different as we've always thought. And as I tried to explain to the woman in the story, if a husband can take the emotional intimacy he feels in the bedroom and share it with his wife in a nonsexual setting, both of their desires will more quickly be met.

TEST YOUR FANTASY LIFE

Choose Y for yes and N for no in response to the following questions:

1. Can you only become sexually aroused if you imagine having sex with someone other than your partner?   Y or N

2. Do you use fantasy to make up for what you believe is missing from your love life?   Y or N

3. When you are troubled or anxious do you tend to turn to sexual fantasies to forget your problems?   Y or N

4. Do your sexual fantasies involve activities that you wouldn't dare do in real life?   Y or N

5. Are your fantasies such that you would never share them with your spouse?   Y or N

6. Do your sexual fantasies occupy a lot of your working hours, taking you away from other activities?   Y or N

7. Do you believe deep down that your fantasies hurt your relationship with your spouse, causing you or her to be unhappy or dissatisfied with the relationship?   Y or N

If you answered yes to any of the previous questions, your fantasy life is not healthy and is undesirable. The more questions you answered yes, the greater a problem your fantasy life is to your sexuality.

6

Why Men Love/Hate Pornography

They catch just about every young boy's eyes sooner or later. High-gloss, colorful, and titillating. They line the magazine racks at every corner newsstand. Some women may take a peek inside, but mostly they appeal to men—even very young men-in-the-making.

Some say it's a rite of passage for teenagers to grow up with them. But the power of the sexual images presented in pornography is so powerful that it always leaves a lasting impression. If it didn't, no one would make a profit. Magazine vendors would switch to selling real estate.

With America showing more skin everywhere, in advertising, movies, on television, and at the beach, voyeurism is becoming the safest sex around. In fact, the marketing of vicarious sex is about the biggest business there is.

Who is the prime target for this business? Males, of course. Who is most harmed? Some would say women are, and to a great extent they are right. But I think it is men. On their behalf, I would agree with Erma Bombeck: "Will someone please notice Madonna so we can get on with our lives!"

The American male has a love/hate relationship with pornography. The love and the hate do not always coexist in the same male. Some men hate it; a lot of men love it. And more than a few love and hate it at the same time. For them it has become an addiction.

Pete is an example of the I love it/I hate it group. He grew up on *Playboy*—saw his first one at age five and hasn't stopped looking since. It had its place of honor on his father's desk, openly and unashamedly displayed. It was a symbol of manhood and authority. He had the right to look at *Playboy*, whether his wife liked it or not.

For many years after his first, shocking look at nude pictures, Pete would sneak into his father's study and page through the magazines. At first the excitement came simply from doing something naughty. But as he grew, he came to experience excitement from the pictures. The nude, gorgeous girls became his friends. His budding sexuality was profoundly influenced. No one told him that the pictures were touched up with an airbrush, flaws removed. He thought all girls looked like that when naked.

At about age twelve, Pete graduated to hard-core magazines—his friend's father was into stronger stuff than *Playboy*. While their parents were at work, the boys would get together to pore over the raunchy pictures. Pete would then go home and masturbate, trying to visualize what he had seen. No sooner had he masturbated than he would feel ashamed of himself.

It wasn't guilt Pete felt—no one in the family knew about his activities. It was shame. The boy was mortified by his lack of control. He was pained at the thought that if others knew what he was doing (apart from his equally guilty friend), they would disown him.

"Love and hate pretty well sum up my feelings about pornography," he told me at our very first session together. "If I only loved it, I wouldn't be here. If I just hated it, I wouldn't be here, either. But here I am."

Why does pornography have a greater attraction to men than women? Women generally hate it.[1] It turns men on, but turns women off. Women respond erotically to touch, sound, smell, relationship, and romance; men to visuals, sounds, and nudity. Women need intimacy for sex and desire pleasure from its whole experience. Men don't need intimacy in quite the same way—the act itself is enough. Men are at greater risk not only of separating sex from love, but of separating sex from real people. Pornography can easily become an impersonal outlet for sex.

Different Effects of Pornography

My first exposure to pornography occurred when I was ten or eleven—late in the Second World War. Soldiers were returning to South Africa

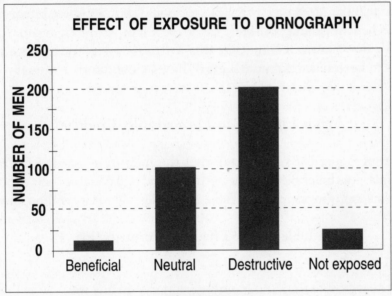

Figure 6.2

One male student later described his reaction to the films as primarily anxiety and embarrassment. They were not sexually arousing. When the class was over, however, and he returned to his apartment, his memories of the movie scenes caused intense excitement. His thoughts were more exciting than the actual images. Erotic material can stimulate private thoughts that later can cause arousal. The effect is a delayed one and sometimes is only acted upon in privacy.

When pornography portrays unequal power relationships, coercive sex, rape (which is not that much different from coercion), violence, or unusual sexual practices, can it be argued that those who watch these materials are not influenced by them? What if, after viewing explicitly erotic images, the viewer has no willing partner available for sex? Who is this excitement likely to be taken out on?

Beyond arousal, there is always a consequence. We cannot dismiss the effects of pornography as inconsequential. While some healthy men might be able to control their use of stimulating material only to enhance their own experience, who knows what long-term secondary effects there may be? Therapists might be able to help dysfunctional couples overcome sexual fears or ignorance with films or books, but are the consequences always beneficial and positive?

We don't know. I would say this with assurance: the average male needs to be very careful in looking at how he uses erotic material.

What Effects Can Pornography Produce?

From Figure 6.2 you will see that the men in my study were overwhelming in their opinion that nothing good had come of their exposure to pornography in their youth. Table 1 provides a summary of their answers.

Table 1: The Effects of Pornography

	Yes	No
Was the exposure to pornography educational in any way?	2%	98%
Was it helpful?	3%	97%
Was its effect neutral?	3%	97%
Was it harmful?	84%	16%
Did you feel it was degrading to women?	80%	20%
Does it promote violence toward women?	58%	42%
Does it degrade sex?	71%	29%
Is pornography addicting in any way?	70%	30%
Does it distort sexuality?	82%	18%
Was it destructive?	71%	29%

The picture here is clear. As men look back later in life on how pornography has influenced them, the overwhelming majority see its influence as negative and perhaps even destructive. "But," some of my readers might protest, "your sample is a very biased sample. It involves men who are mainly married and predominantly religious. Christians have strong negative biases against pornography. So all you are proving is that religious men don't like pornography."

And you are right on all counts. But my opinions about pornography are not shaped only by this group. I have been a therapist to all sorts of men. I have seen the profound effects of pornography on a much larger group than this. Besides, it is not only religious fanatics who are concerned. Professional groups and libertarians are seeing pornography's dangers, too.

A "20/20" program (ABC Television), first aired on January 29, 1993, was a real eyeopener for me. John Stossel was the correspondent and presented a report on the impact of pornography on young people. It nearly knocked Hugh Downs and Barbara Walters off their pedestals.

The program focused on twelve or thirteen male students at Duke University. These were not religious students—just ordinary young men in their early to middle twenties. They were sensible, balanced, and thoughtful young men, clearly not prudes. They had been meeting together for some time, exploring the damaging effects of having grown up on porn. And they had come to believe that their ideas about sex may have been shaped by the sexually explicit pictures they saw as boys. Now they wanted to do something about it.

One student described how when he was quite young, he and another little boy found dozens of *Playboy* and *Penthouse* magazines, along with some more hard-core publications. They took them out, cut out the pictures they liked, and traded them like baseball cards with other kids. They traded blondes for brunettes, kneeling positions for lying-down positions, whatever they wanted. They were only in the third grade, so they didn't know much. But one remembers saying, "These women are mine."

His first sexual experience was dividing up nude women.

What effect do these students see of this early exposure? One said that it "sort of gave me permission to look at women as sexual beings, as only sexual beings." They all agreed that pornography was sex education—but the wrong sort. They weren't debating whether porn was right or not, legal or not, but were simply exploring its impact. And they couldn't have been more honest.

What were some of the messages these young men had learned from the magazines they had perused?

- Women were shown at work, then naked. *The message?* Wherever women are, at their core they are sexual.

- Women were always perfectly formed, beautiful. *The message?* It is these unrealistic features that set the standards for sexuality.

- The magazines repeatedly presented males as being in control. *The message?* Males must push for sex, take control, or else it doesn't happen.

- The hard-core stuff also presented many sexual fantasies as being violent and forceful. *The message?* Pain and sex go together. The more pain, the better the sex.

- Girls (or better still, women) were always ready in these magazines. Just say the word and it's go. *The message?* If your girl (woman) isn't ready at all times there must be something wrong with her.

Talking about the relational effects, the young men described again and again how they had been harmed. Here are some of their stories.

- They went into their first serious dating relationships with a lot of insecurity. The images they had been exposed to were unrealistic. How could they ever measure up?

- Fantasizing and masturbating as much as they did, they had created a powerful sexual reality in the pictures themselves. By a process of conditioning, the pictures had become more reality than reality itself. Women in the pictures didn't have a will of their own. They didn't resist. They didn't talk back. It is much easier to get sex from pictures than from real women.

- The magazines had taught them that women are, in a sense, easy. All it takes is a little persuasive talking. If you push the right buttons anyone will be responsive. *The message?* If a woman says no, she doesn't mean it. Never in any porn magazine or movie does a story end without success for the male.

All the Duke University men interviewed said that the lessons they had learned from pornography had proved destructive when they tried to relate to real women. One said he went through four or five serious relationships, trying to work through the difference between his porn and the real world of love. The magazines hadn't told him how to handle his feelings.

Those who had sexual experiences in college said that in order to climax, they had had to conjure up images from their magazines to do it.

Have they begun to change? Yes, but slowly. At least they're talking about it. They've broken the silence between themselves as men. They're risking being honest. And talking about it will make a difference.

Pornography and the Married Man

After many years of working with both Christian and non-Christian men, I have formed the impression that a lot of married men continue to use pornography as a sexual stimulant after marriage. Having a regular sexual partner doesn't necessarily remove the need for pornography nor for masturbation. Once these habits are established, they continue for a long time.

The Janus Report states that 24 percent to 32 percent of males "actively" masturbate.[6] It is not clear what the percentage is just for married men, but Janus and Janus report that 25 percent of eighteen- to twenty-six-year-olds, 24 percent of twenty-seven- to thirty-eight-year-olds, 8 percent of thirty-nine- to fifty-year-olds, and 21 percent of fifty-one- to sixty-four-year-olds masturbated daily or weekly. Only 5 percent of men preferred masturbation as their method of climax over anything else.

In my study I specifically sought information about masturbating to pornography. My analysis shows that 15.5 percent of married men who are not clergy and 6.8 percent of married clergy, continue to masturbate to pornography while married.

These figures are lower than what I had anticipated out of my clinical experience. Nevertheless, one in six married men, even with a strong religious orientation, still find it necessary to use pornography to stimulate themselves to masturbation.

Why is pornography so popular, even for males who are married and have a ready sexual outlet? Apart from early conditioning to it, one reason is that humans are notoriously curious. A small percentage of men use pornography to satisfy curiosity. A more potent reason is that sex has become dehumanized. It is no longer regarded in many circles as an act between loving, responsible couples, united in a permanent relationship. Sex has become a sport. It invites spectators. And as in all sports, there is a strong desire to improve one's performance. So pornography is used as an aid in becoming better champions.

Finally, porn continues to be popular for married men because sex, both its psychology and its physiology, tends to become habituated to stimulation. With one level of repeated stimulation, sexual excitement weakens. For something to remain pleasurable one must not do it all the time. Novelty is important to all pleasure, including sexual. Many men turn to erotica to restore lost interest or to revitalize a flagging sexual life.

Bobby did that. After being married for ten years sex became boring to him. The novelty wore off. He found himself getting more excitement out of clinching a sale for his business than out of sex. Slowly he began avoiding it.

His wife, however, noticed that things were changing. She had always believed that sex serves an important function for married couples. As she knew it strengthens the bond and gives a reason for couples to stay together. It fosters intimacy and emotional security; it bolsters self-esteem and even provides a tranquilizing effect that reduces tension and anxiety.

So Bobby's wife began to miss these blessings of sex, not just its pleasures. She complained—loud and firm. Something was wrong and they had to work at fixing it, she rightly demanded.

Of course she wanted to go into counseling, but Bobby decided he could fix his problem by just getting turned on through porn. He paid a few visits to sleazy, X-rated movie houses, invested in a few choice home movies and magazines, and declared himself fully alive again. Whenever their "date" came along, he would take a few hours to indulge his porn and get his hormones going.

For a while it seemed to work. But as so often happens, the improvement was short-lived. The films and pictures worked, all right, but transferring the arousal from the pictures or movies to his wife was not always effective.

Bobby became dependent on the erotica. Without it, he couldn't perform. Like a drunken actor who becomes dependent on the freedom that alcohol brings to the acting spirit, Bobby's sexual fire became dependent on the fuel that porn provided. And he had to stoke the fire even hotter each time around. Soon he found himself looking at "S and M" (that's sadomasochism, where pain and suffering are inflicted as part of sexual pleasure). Finally, when he found himself drawn to kiddie porn he sat up with a start. This stuff knows no boundaries, he realized. It is a bottomless pit. It never becomes satisfying.

The road to recovery was slow, very slow, for Bobby. Even today, many years after treatment, he's not so sure he is out of the woods. He believes it wouldn't take much to push him back into a dependence on erotica for sexual arousal.

Breaking the Pornography Obsession

My intention is not to make this book a manual for recovery from sexual hang-ups. However, some comments about how to break a dependency on pornography may be helpful to the reader. What changes are required to break the obsession with pornography? It's important to remind yourself that you have a choice when it comes to behavior. You can break the habit gradually or go cold turkey and stop it all at once. I think cold turkey is best for this addiction. Gradual never works because it keeps the exposure going. So here are some practical suggestions:

- *Pull out and destroy all your porn.* Don't leave anything around, no matter how insignificant you might think it is. Just a little left available will keep you hooked.

- *Change your habits.* Don't go to stores that sell porn. Change the way you go home from work. Avoid places that provoke you sexually. Choose to stay away from temptation.

- *Don't feed your fantasies.* Like pigeons in every European city's central square, your fantasies return only because you feed them. Stop feeding them and, like the pigeons, they will go away. Try to catch yourself whenever you fantasize about some porn; distract your thoughts by choosing to think about something else.

- *Be accountable.* If your partner can handle it, set up a system of accountability with her in which you try to be honest and report your successes and failures. If you know you have to report your actions to your partner, you'll be more vigilant. Changed behavior needs to be celebrated, too, so sharing your successes will help to reinforce them.

If these guidelines don't help you, get professional help from a competent psychotherapist.

Many men turn to pornography to meet needs they're not even aware of. Sometimes it's a need for self-nurturance. Sometimes it's because they are lonely and don't know how to build a more fulfilling relationship. Even married people can feel very cut off and disconnected. Do yourself a favor and get help. Getting at these deeper, unmet needs takes more than self-help. A little insight and practical guidance from a good therapist could save you years of unhappiness and help you to become a more complete person.

You may also want to change your sexual routine. If your problem is sexual boredom, then try having sex less frequently. Having sex too often can take away some of the biological excitement that provides pleasure. Work at being a more romantic partner. Women are different in so many ways. The more you understand their differences, the easier it will be to foster a closer, more romantic, relationship. Flowers, kindness, respect, gentleness, candlelight dinners, and good music are the essential ingredients for romance. It's such a pity that men stop offering these gifts so soon after marriage. Believe me, they never lose their power to bring a more complete fulfillment to the sexual experience of both men and women.

The Dangerous Traps of Repression and Denial

May I offer one final word of caution?

There will be well-meaning readers who will not be able to identify with those men who say that they have struggled unsuccessfully all their lives with their obsession with pornography. Those readers might even say, "Just ask God to deliver you from this battle. It's sin and must be dealt with like all sin. Confess it, repent, and change your ways."

I have seen men take these spiritual steps to find significant release from their lust and longing for porn. Thank God for this. But it doesn't happen every time! I have also known many godly men (and even women) who have prayed with all their might to be released from their obsession, but to no avail. They suffer in great misery, and a few even view sex as God's greatest mistake. Why God helps some men and not others, I don't know.

I do know that lust and pornography (and they are closely linked) can be a powerful prison. In their desperation some men try to resolve their problem with lust and porn by *repressing* their sexuality. They turn themselves off to all forms of stimulation in a sort of emotional castration. Women become impersonal objects.

Whenever these men feel the slightest tinge of sexual arousal they retreat into some religious fervor or spend hours in prayer, all the time repressing their sexual feelings. Husbands have held back their sexuality to such an extent that they have no sexual feelings for their own wives.

This is classical repression, and every psychologist knows how damaging and dangerous it can become. Severely repressed sexual feelings can make such a man a walking time bomb, even if the repression is couched in religious or pious trimmings. This is one of the reasons why so many clergy succumb to sexual temptation (we've seen a bit of an epidemic in this regard in recent years). When you repress sex you don't make it safe. You turn out the light and peril in the dark becomes even more dangerous.

Sexuality must be confronted with courage, not repressed by cowardice. We have to be honest with ourselves before we can build adequate controls over our sexual impulses. I take issue with those who claim that every man can master his lust only by being "delivered" from it. Some are delivered; many are not. For those who are not, it takes hard work with lots of self-honesty and continued vigilance to overcome their passionate sexuality. Their distortion has been learned and programmed deeply into their minds. It takes a lot of unlearning to reverse the process and bring a healthy freedom.

Steer clear of repression as a way of controlling your sexuality, and strive to the utmost in your ability to develop a well-rounded sexual responsiveness. For most men this isn't easy. Real life is too complicated, relationships too demanding, and time too short. To make matters more difficult, real sex is complicated and demanding. But I also know this: In the long run real sex delivers what it promises. Pornography doesn't!

HOW TO BREAK A PORNOGRAPHY ADDICTION

1. Be honest with yourself and acknowledge that you have a problem.

2. Be accountable to another person. Tell someone else you can trust about your addiction.

3. Dispose of all the pornographic material you own. Keep none of it. If you're tempted to rent videos, don't go near a video store of any kind. If you have to, throw away your video rental card.

4. Be patient and resist feeling defeated each time you fail. Your addiction took time to develop, so it will take time to die.

5. Pray about your problem. Depend on God for deliverance and strength. God promises to make a difference in our lives. Allow Him to give you the special strength you need to overcome this battle.

7

Teenage Sexuality

Ann Landers tells the story of a mother who found a collection of nude pictures in a box under her fifteen-year-old son's bed. The mother boasted that she had "cured" her son by pasting the nudes on the living room wall and shaming him.

"That," she crowed, "ended his career as an art collector!"

Ann thought the mother's solution was ingenious and amusing and said so. But she soon found out that a lot of her readers disagreed with her. It wasn't funny, they said. It was just about the most destructive thing any parent could do to an otherwise normal kid going through a normal stage of sexual discovery. So Ann reversed her opinion. Even the best can't be right all the time!

What the mother did was about as cold-blooded and harsh a punishment as anyone could devise. True, the son will never hide his pictures under his bed again. But cured? Of what?

It is not easy in our culture for boys to negotiate the stormy seas of adolescence. The teenage years can be the most miserable passage in many boys' lives. And when you add to the equation insensitive parents, disinterested parents, or parents who have not yet come to terms with their own sexuality, you are likely to create a pretty mixed-up kid.

Discovering Your Body

There is a natural tendency for boys to be very curious about their sexuality. This curiosity starts before puberty and ends at the grave. How this curiosity is dealt with is crucial to the young boy's sexual development.

For a boy, discovering his body in the early years of adolescence can be a strangely frightening experience. A friend of mine, only thirteen years of age at the time, will never forget his discovery.

It was our first year of high school. Teachers thought we should learn to dance. Foxtrot, waltz, slow-step, that sort of thing. It was the slow-step that did it. We could choose whomever we wanted as a partner. Boys lined up on one side, girls the other, in our large school hall. Someone started the record player and the boys ran across, scrambling for the girl of their choice. I chose one I had a crush on, and so did my friend.

We took up our dance positions, hands in all the right places, and started dancing. Slow, slow, quick, slow. My friend held his girl a little too close. The next thing he knew, there was a growing wet patch at the front of his pants. Embarrassed, he fled the scene. As soon as the dance was over I went in search of him. I found him locked in a toilet shivering. He didn't know what had hit him.

His parents hadn't told him a thing. I played doctor and explained about spontaneous emissions, even nocturnal ones. But to this day I suspect he never really understood what had happened. Puberty had arrived with a bang. And even when you've been told what to expect, the first experience of orgasm can blow your mind away.

A boy's first orgasm often happens by accident, in a dream, climbing a rope in gym, or standing next to a girl. It can be embarrassing and is almost certainly unforgettable. Seldom do parents teach how orgasm happens, so in some cases boys experiment with themselves and find out by accident what triggers it. To provide stimulation they turn to visual stimuli. If there are no sexual magazines around, they get caught up paging through encyclopedias or *National Geographic,* intrigued by female nudity. Even a Sears catalog showing female underwear has been known to be a boy's first source of stimulation.

Parents need to understand these first few years of sexuality and do a better job of informing their boys. They must set aside being judgmental or critical. Compassion and empathy can minimize embarrassment and humiliation. Finally, parents should be ready to pour on all the forgiveness they can muster for any mistakes made. This shouldn't just apply to their teenage sons, but to themselves as well. Mistakes will be made; minimizing their damage is an important parenting goal.

Understanding Puberty

Sexual desire which arises during the years of sexual maturity is a physiological law. We don't choose it; it is handed to us. The dawn of this desire coincides with the maturing of the sexual glands and with the development of enough physical mass to support sexual function. Herein, as we will see, is part of the problem. The physiology of sex only needs for the body to be mature. It ignores the maturity of the *mind*.

With improved health and good care, boys are becoming physically mature at earlier and earlier ages while remaining emotionally and mentally immature. Males are given the equipment for sexual performance before their brain is mature enough to control it. And that spells trouble. You may want to review chapter 3 with regard to the age at which boys and girls attain puberty. A few additional points are also worth noting.

- Children who live in cities usually mature a year or so earlier than those who live in the country. The larger the town, the earlier the development and the stronger the drive.

- Heredity is a major factor in both development and sexual drive. Just as physical strength and longevity vary in families, so sexual drive varies from family to family. There is no connection, by the way, between physical strength and sex drive.

- Men and women differ quite markedly in the duration of sexual reproductive ability. The reproductive period is shorter for women than for men but bears no direct relation to the drive for sex. Sexual interests outlast the reproductive period in both men and women.

More Than Animal Instinct

The sexual instinct is under the control of the highest part of the brain, the cortex, which is the part of the brain that learns everything. Sexual expression for the human is only slightly instinctive. Nature gives us a sex drive, but we learn how to direct it. *What* excites the male, *how* it excites, and what *satisfies* this excitation are primarily *taught* to the brain.

By contrast, the behavior of lower forms of life is programmed by instinct. In humans it is tied to feelings, the senses, willpower, ideas, imagination, and thoughts. Unlike animals, we don't need some unique scent to start our juices going. Only the human species is capable of sex at any time. Animals have to wait for a breeding season. The executive organ for sex in humans is the brain, not just the reproductive system.

Why is this important? Because the mind needs to be programmed in the right way. For instance, thoughts can not only stimulate the sex drive, they can inhibit it as well. But not all programming is healthy or natural. Some programming distorts the sexual response, causing an individual to be responsive to the wrong objects. An obvious example of this is the pedophile who is attracted to children.

It is especially important that sexual programming during the pre-puberty and adolescent years be the healthiest possible. The son who collects nude pictures in a box under his bed *may* just be engaging in a natural, curious quest for understanding about the female body. But as we know from our study of pornography and its dangers, pictures, especially the wrong pictures, can program a boy's mind in an unhealthy way.

Teenagers Are Sexual Beings

Our preoccupation with sex in adult life and marriage has caused many to forget that teenagers are sexual beings. Whether adults like it or not, however, teenagers will engage in sexual behavior. Some will just look. Others will have crushes, get involved in petting, masturbating, and in some cases, intercourse. Many parents don't want to face reality. They see every other family's teenager misbehaving sexually but still imagine that "it couldn't happen to our boy."

A recent "Front Page" TV program (Fox TV, November 20, 1993) reported that a school in New Haven, Connecticut, is considering giving condoms to its twelve-year-olds. Twelve-year-olds who should be playing with Barbie dolls and skateboards are demanding condoms: "Give us condoms or else . . . !" they demanded. Some kids reported having sex in the sixth grade. In fact, it is estimated that one-third of eleven-year-olds are now experimenting with sex.

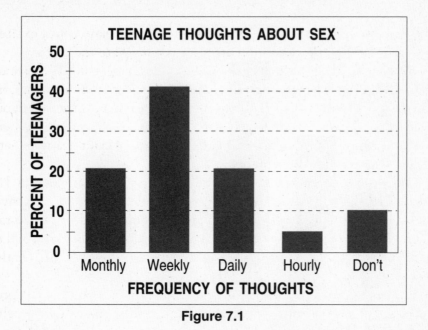

Figure 7.1

Is giving twelve-year-olds condoms the only answer to the dropping age of sexuality? It seems like resignation: "We've given up on you. You're hopeless! We can't seem to teach you any morals or decency, so go ahead and do what you want to do."

One thing is very clear. There are no easy solutions to the problems of teenage sexuality. While the age of puberty continues to drop and parents fail to teach abstinence as a positive alternative, dispensing condoms to young children may be the only other thing schools can do. AIDS is deadly serious business, and teenage pregnancies are rampant.

But is dishing out condoms without even a discussion the only alternative? Girls especially need to know that they are the losers when boys get their satisfaction. If "just say no" is good enough to slow down the drug craze, then why won't it work for the sex craze?

The Nature of Teenage Male Sexuality

How do teenagers experience their sexuality? For instance, how often do teenagers have thoughts about sex? Examining the responses of the males in my sample who were under twenty years of age, I came up with the distribution shown in Figure 7.1. As one would imagine, the average

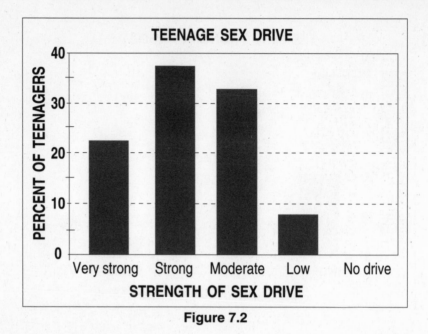

Figure 7.2

teenager thinks about sex several times a week. In contrast, older men think about it several times a day. They've had a lot more practice! Thinking about sex several times a day and several times a week accounts for 63 percent of teenage boys. About 5 percent think about sex several times an hour. What is interesting is that about 10 percent of boys say they never think about sex. What they are probably saying is that sex is not a dominant theme in their thinking. They are definitely in the minority.

How strong do adolescents perceive their sexual drive to be? Figure 7.2 gives the answer. A total of 60 percent of teenagers see their sex drive as either "very strong" or "strong" when compared with their peers. Only 7 percent see it as "low." None reported that they had no drive. So even those teenagers who reported that they don't dwell on sexual thoughts admit that their sex drive exists. Around 32 percent describe it as "moderate."

Our culture generally fails to make adequate provision for boys' sexual drive. I don't just mean dishing out condoms. I mean owning it as a significant force in the development of the teenager and dealing with it maturely and sensibly.

While the entertainment industry continuously caters to adolescent sexuality, moms and dads prefer denial. Unconcerned parents leave their teenager's sexuality to be formed haphazardly. Even good parents don't do

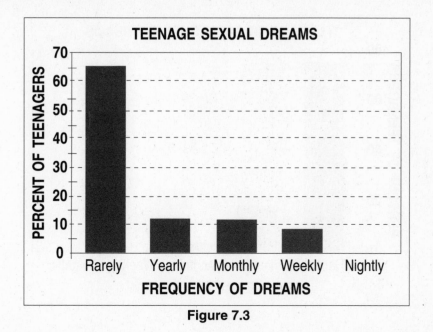

Figure 7.3

very well. They foster repression by indicating that a boy's sexual feelings are not acceptable. This is especially common in religious homes, where a concern for spirituality exists. In any case, every therapist or family counselor will tell you how damaging repression can be.

Research is clear that boys resort to a wide variety of ways to get sexual release and pleasure despite lack of an appropriate outlet.[1] There was a time when boys relied on nocturnal emissions (also called wet dreams) as their major outlet. Not anymore. I asked my teenage male sample how often they had sexual dreams. Figure 7.3 shows the results. Around 66 percent reported they rarely had sexual dreams and 12 percent that they had them monthly. This is less frequently than my adult male sample, 61 percent of whom reported that they rarely had sexual dreams and 21 percent said monthly. I found this to be a most interesting finding, having expected more frequent sexual dreams in teenagers. It appears, however, that teenage boys dream slightly less frequently about sex than adults.

Do teenagers have orgasms in their dreams? Around 18 percent of my total sample reported having orgasms in their dreams yearly while 75 percent reported rarely having orgasms. (See Figure 7.4.)

So where have all the nocturnal emissions gone? The answer is not difficult to discern. Masturbation has taken over what wet dreams used to

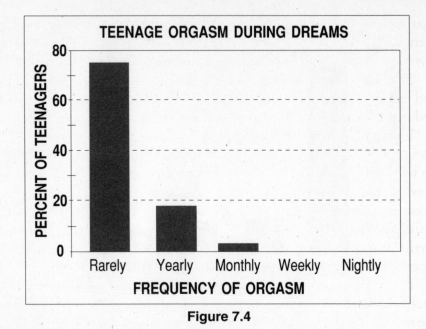

Figure 7.4

accomplish. For the majority of teenage males, it seems that masturbation is the most commonly used release for their built-up sexual tension. Next come petting and sexual intercourse, especially as the teenager gets older.

I did not seek information about intercourse frequencies for teenage boys. This information is readily available from other sources. Janus and Janus, for instance, report that 19 percent of boys report having had sexual intercourse by the age of fourteen. A small percentage had their first intercourse before age ten.[2]

The point is this: sexual desire and ability are occurring at younger and younger ages. The only satisfactory solution, short of finding a way to raise the age of puberty, is to teach all young people that maturity in other areas of their lives is required before they can embark on the sexual adventure. There must be a *period of waiting, a period of abstinence*.

Can ten-, twelve- or even fourteen-year-olds responsibly handle sex? Can they reliably use condoms? Absolutely not. They hardly take care of the car they borrow from you at sixteen, let alone behave responsibly in sex. Adults can barely manage sex. How can immature boys expect to bear this responsibility?

Our society has to rediscover the value of self-control and restraint, teaching it at all ages and levels of society. We also need to stop believing that sexual experimentation during adolescence is a necessary developmental phase for boys. It's time we counted the costs of out-of-control boys and the resulting unwanted teenage pregnancies and abortions.

In some parts of the U.S. 82 percent of teenage males have had full and regular intercourse by age nineteen.[3] And how do secular researchers and sex advocates respond to this information? They say, "Use it or lose it," or "Boys will be boys." An example is *The Janus Report*. It responds to those concerned with the early age at which teenagers are getting caught up with sex by saying that it is a "performance game."[4] The Januses say they can find no scientific data regarding later detrimental repercussions of early sexual activity, so they conclude that the idea that too much sexual activity in early life is damaging to sexuality later on is a "popular myth." Instead, they say, high levels of sexual activity in youth means greater sexual activity in later years.

I can well see why an early start with sex could make us more active in later life. But there *are* numerous detrimental consequences. What about the many girls who are date-raped or impregnated along the way and now suffer from a fear of intercourse? What about the painful experiences of being coerced into sex, hoping to win a boy's love? The overly active sexual male teenager may well continue to be oversexed in later life, but this doesn't mean that no one has been harmed along the way.

Such debates are usually one-sided and consider only the males' perspective. Boys don't have to suffer through an unwanted pregnancy or abortion—they can just "get it off" wherever they want to and then leave the scene. And most parents of these boys are either too embarrassed or too sexually illiterate (by the Januses' own admission) to discuss sex with them before the damage begins.

The Long Waiting Period Distorts Sexuality

As described in chapter 3, there is clear evidence that the age of puberty is continuing to drop. The lower it drops, the longer the waiting period before a young male can expect to have a permanent sexual partner. At the other end, the age at which a young male can reasonably afford to set up a home is rising. A boy who reaches puberty at twelve may not be able to financially marry until he is in his early thirties. This spells trouble for male sexuality. Of all the issues concerning sexuality facing us today this is the most important, yet it is receiving no attention.

It is during this long period of waiting that males are expected to control, even ignore, their sexuality. Now, while I have strongly advocated that boys must learn control, I don't want to minimize the hardship this waiting game imposes on the good teenager. It takes enormous willpower and incredible character to choose to be celibate during this waiting period. It's so much easier to just do what everyone else is doing. One solution is the very common practice of "just living together." Besides the moral dilemma this poses for some religious people, recent research seems to indicate that this does not ensure a more successful marriage. In fact, marriages between couples who have lived together are more likely to fail than those between couples who have not.

It is during this long period of waiting, between puberty and marriage, that most of the distortions of male sexuality are formed. The longer the waiting, the greater the distortions. Even if a male develops a regular sexual partner outside of wedlock, the absence of any long-term commitment has a detrimental effect on the sexual content of the relationship. Having sex with a variety of partners may take care of a man's biological or hormonal needs, but it seldom fosters the development of a whole and healthy sexuality. Commitment is a necessary ingredient in mature love. Passionate love doesn't see the need for it until the morning after.

What are the primary distortions that occur during the long waiting period? Allow me to mention them briefly because they will each be explored in greater detail later.

Teenage boys develop a wrong attitude toward sex. "Sex is pleasure," a teenager once told me, "nothing else." This particular teenager was misbehaving sexually all the time. In fact neighborhood girls were justifiably afraid that he would rape them. Is sex just for pleasure? Our culture and its voice the media seem to think so. Sex's connection to having babies is relegated to nonsignificance.

Another wrong attitude, even more dangerous, says, "Sex is the way I dominate my girls." Sex and the domination of females are closely linked in the masculine mind, and this attitude is created during the long waiting period.

Many male teenagers think of sex as a game of domination. "If a girl says no, you've got to try harder because she doesn't mean it. *Winning* is what sex is all about." Well, this speaker doesn't really mean *winning*. He means *domination*. For him, sex is about control and power, about who rules. This thinking is a major cause of the violence against women that seems to be escalating in these times. It is most commonly expressed in teenage sexuality as date-rape. Violently forcing sex out of a girl can be very exciting for a male because it creates an adrenaline rush. Women, meanwhile, always experience rape as an act of violence, not sex.

Healthy sexual attitudes should include an understanding of sex's role in marriage, procreation, respect for women, and in the appropriateness of restraint and abstinence.

Bad attitudes about these things can be learned, but they also come into being by themselves. They're like weeds. No one I know cultivates weeds—they just grow. Good attitudes, however, have to be cultivated. They are never learned if they are not taught.

Teenage boys learn to misuse fantasy. According to one researcher, about half of teenagers regularly use fantasy with masturbation.[5] I think the percentage is higher than this. Fantasy serves several purposes in adolescence:

- It creates and supports sexual arousal; it adds pleasure to sexual activity.

- It serves as a substitute for the real thing (or person) not yet available.

- It rehearses later sexual experiences and provides a safe outlet for sexual experimentation.

But is it safe? My clinical experience teaches me that it easily gets out of control. Let me illustrate.

An older teenage boy I was counseling developed a crush on a certain girl. He had met her at a party. She seemed friendly, so he imagined she had a crush on him, too. Later at the party she told him she wasn't interested in him.

When he got home later that night and tried to go to sleep he found himself fantasizing that he had won her over. This started a pattern of regular fantasizing about her, and in the fantasies she was putty in his hands.

Slowly his fantasies began to distort his reality. He wasn't sure where reality ended and fantasy began. Several times he tried to call her only to have her hang up on him. When he tried to talk to her in person, she rebuffed him. But he ignored her rebuffs and kept coming back. He sat in his truck on the street opposite her house for hours on end waiting to get a glimpse of her comings and goings.

At night he fed his fantasies. He was her hero. She begged for his attention. She even pleaded with him to give her sex. One day he tried to act out one of his fantasies by grabbing her and pushing her into the passenger seat of his truck. The police were called, charges were leveled against him, and his parents finally realized that they had a problem on their hands. So they brought him to me.

Fantasy is only healthy if it occurs in a mature mind, a mind that can constantly check in with reality. Teenagers who learn to fantasize before they are capable of adequately testing reality often confuse the two. Some never learn to tell the difference! Even if they do, real life and real sex with a real person never quite measure up to their visions. Fantasies set us up to expect more than is reasonable.

Teenage boys develop sexual fetishes or "preferences." Fetishism is a form of sexual arousal attached to an object or body part that is not primarily sexual in nature. Fetishes might include women's shoes or underwear. Many objects can take on sexual significance, including leather, rubber, silk, or fur. What determines whether an object takes on the qualities of a fetish? We don't know. It has to be an object connected in some way with women or one that has a sensual feel about it, like silk or fur. Teenagers (and eventually men) derive strong sexual arousal from these objects. They collect them, play with them, wear them, and almost always masturbate with them.

The fetish is not just a symbolic substitute for its owner. In other words, real fetishists don't resort to a woman's item of clothing because there is no woman available. They prefer it to the real thing. A fetish takes on a life of its own because it is safe, silent, cooperative, tranquil, and can even be harmed without consequence. Therefore, someone who is into leather as a fetish might cut and slash it for sexual excitement.

Not all fetishists go to this extreme. And there is a more subtle form of fetishism that develops in all males. We may not even think of it as such, but I would like to explain it in these terms so as to help men understand what they are doing.

I have always been fascinated with how and why men become attached to certain parts of the female anatomy. These take on sexual significance even when they are not in and of themselves sexual in nature—the shape of legs, buttocks, breasts, and so forth. These parts of the female anatomy are certainly not seen in sexual terms in other cultures to the same extent they are in ours.

But there are other subtle fetishes that normal men develop to such objects as high-heeled shoes, dark stockings, a preferred hair color or style, and so on. I know of several marriages that nearly ended in divorce because the husband demanded that his wife have a certain color of hair or hair style. In one case it turned out that the style and color he was wanting was the same his mother wore. The gentleman changed his tune quickly when he finally discovered the connection.

Minor fetishes or preferences are formed primarily during the adolescent years. One man I knew stole a pair of black panties from his older cousin when he was only thirteen. He didn't steal them because they were black or particularly sexy, but simply because the young woman had left it behind when she had stayed with his family during a visit. She was attractive and the panties were a part of her.

The young boy kept the black panties hidden for a few weeks, then took them out to examine them. He became excited, and for some time afterward used them for self-stimulation. Just having his genitals touch the panties excited him to orgasm. From that day on he was hooked on black panties. Nothing else excited him, much to his wife's dismay early in their marriage. She finally refused to wear black panties all the time.

Such early imprinting of a sexual preference is difficult to change if it is left unchallenged. This is why teenagers need to be encouraged to talk with a trusted older person, preferably a father, about their sexual feelings and secret experiences. Unfortunately, it takes a healthy father to be able to address these ticklish and very personal issues honestly and openly. Some fathers may need to seriously consider getting help for themselves *before* their sons reach the teenage years.

Teenagers develop "lovemaps." A "lovemap" is a specifically internalized map of what does and what does not cause sexual arousal. The phrase was coined by Dr. John Money.[6] As boys become aware of their sexual feelings they notice that they are more likely to become aroused by specific types of people. Others have little or no sexual attraction to them.

What causes this selectivity in sexual attraction to develop? How important is it? Clearly it is learned. I doubt if there is a gene that says, "only feel attracted to brunettes, height five-foot-six, dark eyes, and lips that curl at the end." Generally, we are attracted to whatever is most familiar to us. Ethnic groups often feel attracted to their own characteristics, blondes to blondes, and so forth.

I think that this familiarity factor also operates to attract us to people who resemble our own features. When my wife and I were dating, many people thought we were brother and sister. We had many similar physical characteristics, and that's why we were attracted to each other. Familiar habits and behaviors also attract couples together. Later, when they've lived together for a long time they become even more alike.

Lovemaps become fixed in adolescence, and if a teenager is exposed to a wide variety of friends, his lovemap will broaden. Too narrow a lovemap often means that a young adult can never find a partner that suits him. He delays courting and marriage and may even never get married, waiting for the right person to come along. Narrow lovemaps also foster ethnic stereotypes and prejudices.

A broad lovemap makes for greater satisfaction in relationships. One can love and accept a greater breadth of available partners. There is a greater level of acceptance and less forcing of one's partner into a particular mold of preference. In the final analysis, love must foster acceptance of who the partner is, warts and all. The greater the acceptance, the more easily passionate love can mature into compassionate love—the love that lasts. Even this distinction is something that teenagers can be taught.

What Worries Teenage Boys Today?

The long period of waiting while the sexual hormones rage like a firestorm causes many teenagers to become anxious. One of the reasons why the Netherlands is praised for having the lowest teenage pregnancy rate in the Western world (about one in one hundred teenagers) is because confidential information and counseling services are readily available.

When teenagers can talk about their sexual problems they stay healthier.

What are the most frequently asked, worrisome questions that teenage boys are least likely to ask their parents? Here are a few of them:

1. **Why do I get an erection when I don't want to have one?**
   You may be sitting at the dinner table where the conversation is about anything but sex. Suddenly you feel an erection. You can't explain it. It's time to get up and move from the table but you don't dare because someone might see your bulge. You stay seated for as long as possible, but it doesn't go away. The more you think about it, the more you can't get rid of it. So you make some excuse to stay seated and feel like an idiot.

   Boys need to know that during the early stages of sexual maturing, and even later, spontaneous erections can occur. You don't have to be consciously thinking about sex (consciously, that is), yet it happens. A full bladder can trigger it. Tight pants or accidental friction can also do it. The best way to deal with it is to ignore it. A boy should never be made to feel shame or embarrassment because he has an erection. There's nothing he can do to stop it.

2. **Is my penis too small?** Every boy wonders about the size of his penis, usually about whether it is too small. Sometimes it is the opposite. Either way, the worry causes them to become very self-conscious. They avoid undressing with other boys on social occasions where they are likely to be seen. They hide their nudity, don't want to go to a public toilet, and so on. Eventually, they become preoccupied with checking out the size of other boys. They may get teased about being a peeping Tom or worry about whether they are gay or not.

   I can remember very well this stage during high school. I was playing rugby against a team in another town, worrying about the communal shower after the game. I knew boys would be running around naked flicking towels at each other and playing the fool, partly to conceal the awkward feelings of being naked in front of each other. But what if just one boy said something about your private part? Of course you'd respond in anger, lashing out as if your deepest secret had been uncovered. How I dreaded those showers—totally humiliating!

How does one deal with this question? Prepubescent boys don't ask about their penis size for reasons of sex but simply because they are being teased. You reassure the boy that the other boys are just self-conscious themselves, teasing to draw attention away from their own embarrassment.

If the teenager's friends are teasing the boy unmercifully, then perhaps the family should consider changing the boy's environment or friends. There's little to be done in direct confrontation with the troublemakers; it would only make matters worse. Excessive teasing can leave permanent scars that are difficult to eradicate. Drastic action may be needed.

By the way, if the boy is older a parent should explain that successful intercourse has nothing to do with size. Reassurance, particularly in the face of continual harassment, may need to be repeated often.

3. ***Am I abnormal if I remain a virgin?*** I am convinced that many teenage boys seek out a sexual experience because of peer pressure. They want to be seen to be one of the boys. Boys lie, boast, and exaggerate about their sexual exploits. So gullible teenagers begin to feel left out or ostracized.

If they don't feel ready for sex or are a little afraid of it, they may begin to feel that something is wrong with them. That is the time for parents to reinforce the belief that it is quite normal and highly desirable to refrain from excessive petting or full-blown intercourse until marriage. Without this encouragement, young boys may feel pressured into a premature sexual encounter that could be disastrous for them.

It is almost always a disappointing experience to have intercourse before a person is ready for it. I've encountered several men who have been totally put off by a bad experience. Sex is for adults. It is too perilous to be played with by youngsters.

I am totally opposed to teenagers having sexual intercourse. I didn't and most of my buddies didn't. My convictions have nothing to do with my religious beliefs, and I am certainly not a prude. They are an outcome of my many years of observation as a psychologist.

Teenage boys are too young and teenage girls are too vulnerable to be playing at a game that can have such lifelong repercussions. Most teenagers will never be able to use contraception responsibly—they are too impulsive. The high rate of teenage pregnancy shouts this message at us. Teenage pregnancy is unsound medically, psychologically, socially, and morally. So if teenage pregnancy is undesirable, then the behavior that causes it must be unsound also.

Teenagers don't want to hear adult opinions and certainly don't ask permission to have sex. This violates their right to be autonomous. Parents, however, can exert a positive influence. They can gently and calmly teach the virtues of waiting, placing a high value on teenage virginity for both boys and girls.

4. *Am I abnormal if I have sexual thoughts about people I know?* Teenagers need to understand that during the early years of sexual development their sexual desire may be unattached, roaming far and wide, searching for an object" to atach itself to. Even family members are included in this early searching, as well as older women.

Slowly as the teenager matures, he will learn to focus his sexual desire on a specific person. Usually it is someone about his own age and someone who fits his own interests. At this point he learns to inhibit sexual feelings toward family members. And eventually he learns to focus his sexual desires on his partner, excluding all others. This is the beauty of human sexuality. It can confine itself to the one we love.

But for the teenager still in the formative stage, sexual thoughts and desires can range far and wide. Parents should be willing to discuss and explain this with a matter-of-fact attitude and put their young teenager out of his misery.

5. *Am I masturbating too much?* Most boys have no idea what normal is when it comes to masturbation because they seldom discuss it between themselves. Each one feels

that his experience is extraordinary, even abnormal. Invariably, they worry that something may be wrong, and they become anxious about unnecessary or even very normal experiences.

Let us get an important fact straight here. Nearly all teenagers masturbate. For the majority of them, masturbation itself will have no long-term negative consequences. There is a problem, however, with those who do it to excess. What is excessive? I would define excessive as several times a day over a protracted period of time. Some boys may masturbate more than once a day for a short period of time, then return to a less intense pattern.

There are many reasons for excessive masturbation:

- *Severe anxiety.* Sexual arousal and the relief masturbation brings can serve as a form of tranquilizer.

- *Too much sexual stimulation in his environment.* This state of affairs is often seen in lower economic environments or cramped living quarters where a single mother who has a boyfriend is engaging in frequent sex. The teenager is then exposed too readily to this activity. His level of sexual interest is raised too high. Such a boy will be tempted to masturbate often.

- *Unmet emotional needs.* He may be craving maternal or paternal love and this craving for intimacy is being transformed into sexual needs that he can satisfy himself.

- A *powerful flow of sex hormones.* The sexual drive varies from male to male, and there is often a strong genetic reason for this.

Whatever the reason, the boy who masturbates excessively needs to learn how to control this behavior—without guilt. Matter-of-fact, unemotional, and noncondemnatory counseling works best. And it's more effectively done by an impartial professional counselor, not by a parent who may be uncomfortable talking about masturbation.

Normal Teenage Masturbation

How often do normal boys masturbate? Almost all (96 percent) of the males under age twenty in my sample masturbate regularly. The average number of times per month was fourteen, which compares closely with my total sample of men, mostly married, who averaged thirteen times per month. So teenagers really don't masturbate more frequently than older males.

The pattern changes every little with age. Janus reports that 24 percent of males under age twenty-six masturbate daily or several times a week. From age twenty-seven to thirty-eight it is 28 percent; from thirty-nine to fifty it is 23 percent; over fifty, 32 percent. It seems that the habit is established quite early and is continued throughout life.

Much of our modern-day attitudes toward masturbation stem from our Judeo-Christian ethic and history. Jewish tradition emphasized that a man was not to waste his seed. (See Leviticus 15:16–18.) The sin of Onan described in Genesis 38:8–10 was really the sin of interrupting coitus. He refused to obey the law that he was to take his dead brother's wife as his own.

Early Christian practice warned against masturbation. It is hard to believe that just over a hundred years ago the recommended cure for masturbation was castration! Today most respectable researchers say that self-exploration and manipulation is a common form of sexual development. As I see it, the problem is not so much with the self-stimulation as it is with what accompanies it, namely the use of pornography and fantasy.

Masturbation is a controversial topic in many quarters. All I would like to say here is that nothing is gained by increasing a teenager's guilt over his masturbation. No doubt there are a few teenagers who masturbate to excess, but they are in the minority. Boys should be taught matter-of-fact self-control.

While masturbation fulfills an urgent need in adolescents for relieving sexual tension, the interplay of guilt and pleasure can be quite damaging. So some advocate that the solution to the problem of masturbation is simply to remove all taboos against it—let boys be boys and do whatever they want to do.

Is it this simple? Boys are masturbating earlier, are being exposed at younger and younger ages to more and more distorted views of sex through the media and are therefore masturbating more frequently. Males are becoming more and more dependent on porn to sustain their sexual habits. And I, among many psychotherapists, am seeing an increasing number of married men who are saying, "I'd rather just go off by myself with a sexy video or some magazines and take care of myself. Sex is just too complicated, demanding, and not really as great as my private self-stimulation." In the long run this is hardly conducive to building strong marriages and harmonious sexual relationships.

A teenager's early exposure to erotica should therefore be controlled, even eliminated. This is a delicate assignment. As a parent, you might personally condemn pornography, yet you must be careful not to condemn your teenage son for either having an interest in it or in having used it in some way. A healthy sexuality is shaped by positive instruction, not by judgment and condemnation.

Frank, open discussions are the best. And a total ban on masturbation will never be successful or possible. But an honest acceptance of its limitations and hazards, especially when paired with fantasy and porn, is reasonable and workable. If teenage young men can come to understand that the excessive use of masturbation for sexual release can lead to distortions in later life, they might choose to develop the self-discipline to control it. This is a narrow path, I know, although it isn't as narrow as some would like it to be. But I believe it is workable, especially when applied with love, acceptance, and an extra measure of parental wisdom.

COMMON ADOLESCENT SEXUAL MYTHS

1. *Having sex produces instant adulthood.* Many teenagers come to believe that sex is an adult initiation rite. Not only is this idea false, but early sex can damage a teenager's sexuality. It may produce a pregnancy, and the sex itself can even be extremely disappointing.

2. *Having sex is an expression of being in love.* The belief that if you're in love you must have sex pushes many teenagers into premature intercourse. Love does not need sex for proof. Furthermore, having sex with someone will not increase the likelihood that he or she will love you more.

3. *When she says no, she means yes.* Promoted by pornography, this idea lies behind most of what happens in date-rape. Boys just don't understand how girls function in the area of sex and need to be taught how they are different. When girls say no, they mean it.

4. *You can't get pregnant just by doing it once.* Boys want to believe this. Many are totally ignorant about menstrual periods and when a girl is fertile. Because some boys have previously had unprotected sex without causing a pregnancy they spread the idea that it's not so easy to make a girl pregnant. It even adds an element of risk to sex that makes it more exciting. The truth is, it only takes one time to make a baby.

5. *Condoms aren't used by real men.* Younger boys listen to the older boys talk about how condoms decrease pleasure, so they think they must avoid them. There is a culture among boys that works against using condoms. This is the greatest obstacle against advocating protected sex rather than abstinence. We will never teach mere children the proper use of protection. They're too young to take this responsibility.

8

Sex and the Married Man

Most men long for a loving, intimate, exclusive relationship with a woman. Contrary to the stereotype of men who reject commitment and dread being tied down, there is a craving in men for someone to be a special partner. Naturally, marriage provides the best opportunity for fulfilling this need.

Throughout this book I have examined the sexuality of the male, with special emphasis on how to create a healthy sexuality that favors long-term relationships. It should be clear by now that any distortion of the male sex drive increases the possibility of failed marriage. Inability to work out a compatible sexual relationship is, in my experience, the most common cause of marital conflict and breakup. Sometimes the fault lies with the wife. Sometimes it lies with the husband. My concern here is to assess what contribution the male's sexual experiences make toward marital difficulties.

The sample of males I studied is comprised mainly of married men. The length of their marriages is depicted in Figure 8.1. The men I see in psychotherapy are also primarily married men. Staying married is the greatest challenge facing good men today. Why? Because something has gone terribly wrong with the institution of marriage.

Divorce statistics are staggering. Even more alarming is the dramatic increase in divorce among groups that traditionally have had a high view

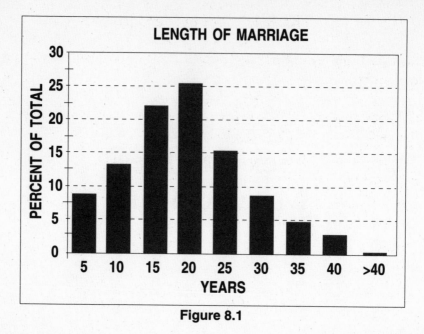

Figure 8.1

of marriage—clergy, for instance. It is becoming increasingly common-place for them to divorce.

It is not always the husband's doing; sometimes the wife throws in the towel. Either she can't take the unhappiness of their marriage or she resents the unusual demands that work places on a marriage. On a few occasions she has taken up with another man or she feels unable to reestablish trust in a husband who has been unfaithful.

But there is a deeper reason why marriage is in trouble today. Couples do not seem to be able to move beyond the romantic stage of love to the deeper love that forms the foundation for long-term relationships. I recall a study several years ago where about six hundred married couples were asked the question, "Do you love your spouse?" Only about 11 percent could answer unhesitatingly, "Yes."

What are the roots of this dismal situation? I am sure there are many causes. For one thing, romantic love seems to hide all the flaws until after the knot is tied. Failure to allow love to mature is another cause. But the problem I want to focus on here, given the topic of this book, is the sexual one. Sex either makes or breaks a marriage, and more often than not it breaks it.

The Role of Sex in Marriage

Let me begin by stating, as clearly as I can, what I believe to be the role of sex in marriage:

- Sex strengthens the bond between man and wife. A satisfying sexual relationship helps to keep a couple together.

- Sex fosters the growth of intimacy (a special type of friendship) in the relationship.

- Sex helps to provide a special privateness that excludes all others from the relationship.

- Sex overcomes many conflicts and helps a couple to come back together whenever there is a rift.

- Sex serves to reduce stress and anxiety by providing a special time of togetherness and a release of tension.

- Sex can become a wonderful way of expressing love between a couple.

- The pleasure of sex provides a shared experience, even when not much else is shared in common in a relationship.

- Sex provides a special sense of emotional security that helps to create a sense of well-being and happiness.

These are all positive benefits that help to strengthen a marriage. But is everything about sex always positive? No it isn't. Sometimes sex or the withholding of it is used to punish a partner. Sexual frustration can cause a great deal of hostility in an unfulfilled partner. And when sex is used to express hostility or to manipulate a partner it has stopped being beneficial. It may even be destructive.

Essential to a satisfactory sexual relationship is an atmosphere of mutual caring, friendliness, openness, sharing of feelings, and commitment. There must be mutual tolerance for shortcomings, a spirit of forgiveness, mutual concern, trust, and freedom from fear. In short, there must be love.

Without love, sex has the potential to become a monster. While I could say a lot about the female's contribution and unique way of providing this

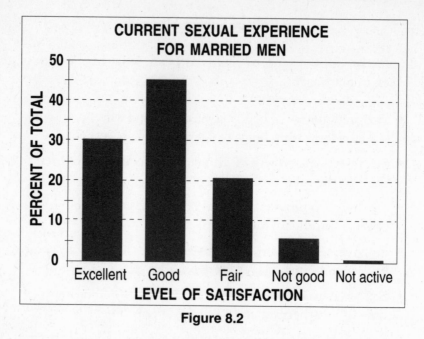

Figure 8.2

love, my focus here is on the male. The male's sexuality, as I have tried to show several times thus far, is often misunderstood both by males and females. I trust that my discussion here will bring some clarification. (If you aren't interested in survey statistics about married men, sex, and masturbation, you may want to skip to "Is Masturbation Helpful to a Marriage?" later in the chapter.)

How Satisfied are Men with Sex?

My sample of married men shows a remarkably high level of satisfaction with their current sexual experience, at least higher than I expected. Figure 8.2 presents the distribution of married males according to their degree of satisfaction. The question I posed was this: "How would you rate your current sexual experience?" The choices ranged from "excellent" to "not active."

Almost three out of four (72 percent) of the men rated their current sexual experience as either excellent or good; 27 percent said it was fair or not good. This means that about two out of three of the men surveyed are really quite satisfied with their sexual lives. They may not be getting the level of satisfaction as they desire, but overall it is high.

Nearly one out of three married men, however, reported that it is only fair or not good. This group constitutes the most dissatisfied of married men. Given that the divorce rate is about one out of two marriages, having one in three married men dissatisfied with their sexual lives doesn't bode well for marital stability.

Perhaps even more telling than the statistics were the comments men wrote on their questionnaires. Some talked about how personal conflicts got in the way of their sexual life. Others commented about the sexual unresponsiveness of their wives. They bemoaned the fact that as girls, their wives were taught to dislike sex. A few spoke of their wives being seriously ill or incapacitated. The overall feeling I got from these written responses was one of profound sadness and regret that marriage had not been more satisfying. The comments were very moving.

The men that wrote these things were by no means looking for an excuse to get out of their marriages. They spoke of staying in for reasons other than sex—companionship, shared life mission, and so forth. Nevertheless, they certainly felt that something was seriously lacking in their sexual lives.

Reasons Why Sexual Needs Were Not Being Met

Even if a married man rates his current sexual experience as excellent or good, it doesn't mean he is getting sufficient sex to feed his biological or psychological needs. Most men I know would prefer to have sex more often than they do. So I asked my sample the question, "Do you feel that your sexual needs are being met?" Choices included always, often, sometimes, rarely and never.

Figure 8.3 presents the results. Around 69 percent said that their sexual needs were being met always or often. The rest (31 percent), however, said that their needs were either only sometimes, rarely, or never. This means that about one in three married men complains of some dissatisfaction about having his sexual needs being met; one in twelve has a major complaint about his sexual needs not being met.

To gain further insight, I asked my sample the question, "What *mostly* prevents you from having your sexual needs met?" The choices included,

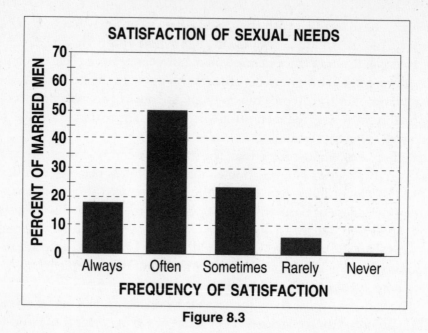

Figure 8.3

my partner is not ready, my partner is unavailable, I am not ready, I am not interested, and other. I included "other" in the event that none of the afore-mentioned categories quite captured the main reason. Figure 8.4 shows the percentage of married men that answered yes to each of these categories.

By far the most common reason that married men gave for not hav-ing their sexual needs met was that their *partner is not ready* for sex at the same time they are. Around 63 percent of the men gave this as the major reason. Only 3 percent said *they (as husbands) were not ready.* Another 3 percent reported that they were not interested in sex. Around 19 percent said their partner was not available. I take this to mean that their partner was either sick, absent, or incapacitated in some way.

Two-thirds of married men, therefore, complained of insufficient sex because their partner was not ready, and my clinical work supports this. The male's need for sex cycles two or three times faster than that of the female's need.

There are probably several reasons for this. Some experts have argued that the male's physiology is designed to be more aggressive about sex.[1] The male is created to be the initiator. We know that men are usually ready for sex. Meanwhile, the female body goes through a readiness cycle tied to reproduction. She is not always responsive.

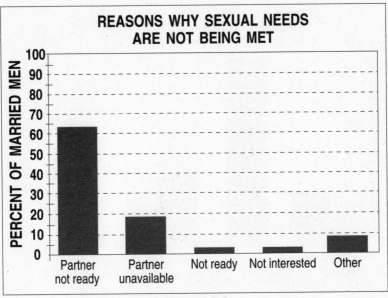

Figure 8.4

This inequality in readiness between the sexes should really be seen as natural; however, it causes much discord in most marriages. Female sexuality is as vexing for men as male sexuality is for women.

There are other differences. First, sexuality in women appears to awaken more spontaneously and makes masturbation in young girls less necessary than in boys.[2] Women do not, as a rule, find masturbation, by itself, as satisfying as men.

A second difference between the sexes is in the male's desperate need for orgasm. In men the drive toward orgasm is everything. It totally consumes them. Sexual arousal that does not culminate in orgasm is extremely frustrating—even anger producing—as many wives know.

For the female, orgasm is not so urgent or necessary. They have nothing to release. After bearing several children, many women even lose interest in orgasm. And when they don't need or enjoy orgasm, they neither need nor enjoy sexual intercourse.

This problem assumes even greater seriousness in marriages whenever a wife has never learned how to trigger an orgasm. About one-third of married women appear to fall into this category. Without the pleasure of orgasm, intercourse becomes an unpleasant and even hated chore. Some avoid it at all costs. Others try to delay the interval between intercourse as long as

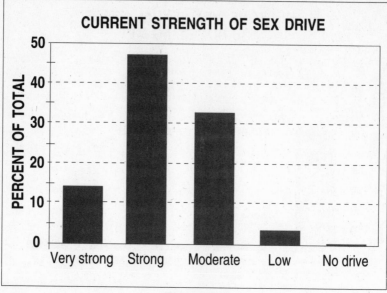

Figure 8.5

possible. Every counselor and therapist encounters this problem in marriages on a daily basis and knows how difficult it is to resolve. Professional help is almost always necessary. Fortunately there are ways to help a woman achieve orgasm or at least to find deep satisfaction in sexual intercourse.

There is yet another reason for the disparity between the sexes in enjoyment of sex. The high incidence of child sexual abuse in girls (some put it between 25 percent and 50 percent of the female population) is often a reason why sex is not enjoyable for these women. Everyone, male or female, who has been sexually abused as a child suffers from some consequence. Unresolved fears and distorted beliefs often act to inhibit the sexual response.

Finally, for most women these days, life is more stressful and fatiguing than it is for men. Working full-time, taking care of the house, raising the kids, feeding the family, walking the dog, pulling the weeds, washing the clothes, and sometimes even paying the bills—these don't leave a lot of energy for sex. Add to all of these factors the poor sexual technique of many husbands and women are not very interested—for good reason.

Men who want a better sex life not only need to learn how to be better lovers, but also how to carry the emotional and physical burden of homemaking and child-rearing. To put it more bluntly: many men only have themselves to blame for their low sexual satisfaction.

Strength of Sex Drive

To assess the current strength of the sex drive in each member of my sample I posed the question, "At present my sex drive is . . . ." Choices ranged from "very strong" to "feel no sex drive." Figure 8.5 presents the results. About 15 percent of the men reported that their sex drive was very strong (one man in six); 47 percent said that it was strong; and 33 percent that it was moderate. Strong to moderate, therefore, accounts for about 80 percent of the men or about four out of five men. Only 5 percent reported a low or nonexistent sex drive.

Clearly the male sex drive is a significant force. But does it always remain this strong? One would expect that as a male ages, the strength of the drive diminishes. Analyzing those who rated their drive as very strong and strong, and looking at the relative percentages for each ten-year age group, I came up with 66.5 percent of men below thirty years of age who rated themselves as being very strong or strong in their sex drive. In comparison, 67.4 percent of the thirty- to forty-year age group saw themselves in this category, while 75 percent of the forties and fifties said the same. It is only when we come to the over-fifties group that this percentage begins to drop down to 41 percent. If anything, then, men see the sex drive as increasing up to age fifty and then only starting to decline.

Where does the sex drive go? It seems to shift down to moderate. Whereas there are 30 percent moderates in the under thirties, 25 percent in the thirties to forties, 31 percent in the forties to fifties, the figure climbs to 43 percent in the fifties to sixties, and 71 percent in the over-sixties age group. So the "strong" and "very strong" move down to being just "moderate." The sex drive cools a little after age fifty, but not a whole lot. In any case, it doesn't go away. And that means its various manifestations need to be considered, particularly in the context of marriage.

Sexual Distractions for the Married Male

One of the greatest struggles every married male has is with his inborn, hormonally pressured interests in sex beyond the marriage. I call these "sexual distractions."

A husband may love his wife very dearly. He may be extremely satisfied with the sexual encounters in his marriage. And then when walking down

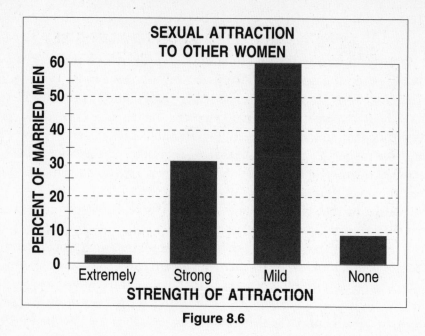

Figure 8.6

the street, riding the bus or commuter train, stopping alongside another car on a busy freeway, or even just sitting on a park bench reading a magazine, his thoughts turn to other women. He sees someone walking by. Attractive. He wonders about her sexuality. He undresses her in his imagination. He entertains fantasies of a sexual rendezvous or being ravaged by her.

This is a good man. "I love my wife," he says to himself. "Why do I think about women this way?"

Men, on the whole, are morally less upright than women. It's a fact, and it doesn't matter how religious they are. If a male has been programmed with a lot of fantasy in adolescence, then he will continue to use fantasy as a sexual escape, no matter how satisfied he is sexually in his marriage. Conscience will have little effect in controlling it.

To get at these issues I posed several questions to my rather conservative, religious sample of good men. First, I asked about their sexual attraction to other women and how strong this attraction is. Figure 8.6 shows the distribution. About 33 percent, or one in three, married, morally upright and good men acknowledged that they were either *extremely* or *strongly* attracted to women other than their wives.

Many men are bothered by the fact that they feel attracted to pretty women. The fact is, men notice attractive women, and they'd have to be

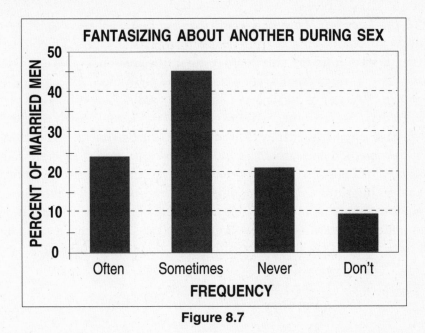

Figure 8.7

blind and brain damaged not to. No immorality is implied just because a man notices a pretty woman.

But the wording of my question and its context gets at a deeper issue. One in three married men is *strongly* attracted, and this attraction is in a sexual way. They don't necessarily do anything about it. They don't act out their attraction. They certainly don't leave their marriages or become unfaithful. But married men *do* experience sexual attraction toward other women. And this attraction is the beginning of lust—a word so old-fashioned that one hesitates to use it.

Men are very conscious of their propensity for lust, which is why it has always been considered to be one of the seven deadly sins. They are conscious of their roving eyes and feel more hypocritical than women in regard to their sexuality. Many wives know this but don't want to hear or talk about it.

Clergy, priests, and rabbis are not particularly exempt. If anything, they struggle with these urges more so than ordinary men. They dare not talk to their wives about it. Women cannot understand why, if their husbands really love them, they would think of other women. So men feel misunderstood, condemned, and even despised.[3] They withdraw into themselves and avoid sharing such intimate, dark secrets that could jeopardize their marital happiness.

Only 7 percent of my sample said they felt no sexual attraction toward other women. Allowing for the 3 percent or 4 percent who also reported no sexual drive or interests, this figure seems quite a reasonably accurate estimate. One in thirteen men are not attracted to women other than their spouse. For the rest of the male population, including deeply religious men, the sex drive is generalized to all women and not focused solely on a wife.

I have already mentioned in another context that this is part of a larger problem, namely, that *all males need to learn sexual discipline and self-control.* Our brains, with appropriate training, can learn how to inhibit sexual feelings in inappropriate directions. For instance, I feel no sexual arousal to family members outside of my wife. This is the wonder of my brain. It can learn where my sex should be focused and where it shouldn't. I'll have more to say about this in the final chapter of this book.

Fantasy and the Married Man

How often do married men fantasize about having sex with another woman, especially during their own masturbation or sex? Figure 8.7 shows the frequency. "Often" accounts for 25 percent of men, while "sometimes" accounts for 45 percent. Around 70 percent of the men, then, nearly three out of four, at least sometimes fantasize about having sex with someone else while having a sexual experience themselves. Only 9 percent said they *don't fantasize*, and 21 percent that they *never fantasize about someone else.* Presumably, if they do fantasize, it is about their own partner.

This is shown in Figure 8.8, which depicts the focus of sexual fantasies. Most of the men in my sample (47 percent) fantasize about their own partner. They may do this during intercourse, but mainly, I suspect, during masturbation.

The next most common person for sexual fantasies is a friend (18 percent), a fantasy person (14 percent), and then a total stranger (12 percent). The stranger is presumably someone they have seen in a movie or just talked to on the street.

My clinical experience indicates that men seldom stick with one person in their sexual fantasies. They switch their focus depending on circumstance, level of arousal, recent exposure to an attractive woman, and so forth. In any case, men do fantasize.

Does this fantasy world actually include having sex with another woman? Figure 8.9 shows that 59 percent of the men include actual sex

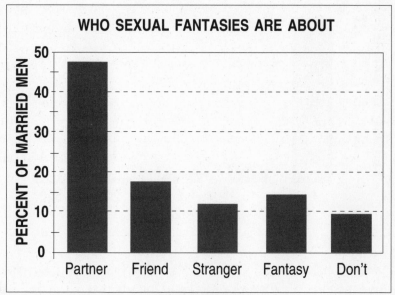

Figure 8.8

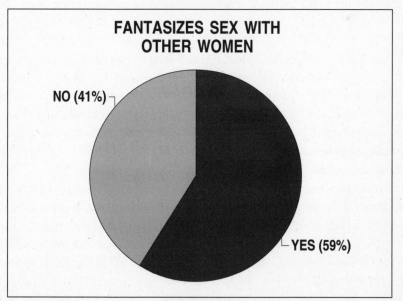

Figure 8.9

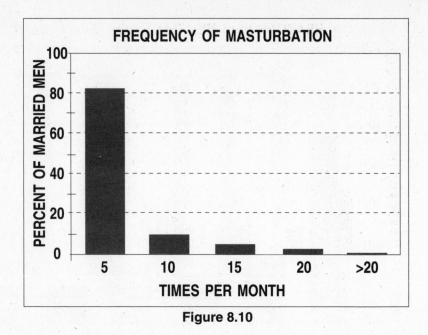

Figure 8.10

with someone else in their fantasies. That's nearly two out of three men. The remaining 41 percent say they don't. This doesn't mean that they have never done it, just that they don't do it on a regular basis.

Do Married Men Masturbate?

This now brings me to one of the most vexing and complicated issues regarding the sexual activity of married men, namely, their continued use of masturbation. I have counseled more men troubled by this than any other sexual problem. In some circles it is not considered to be a problem; in my circles, it is.

First of all, let us examine what percentage of married men are currently masturbating. In my sample it is 61 percent—three out of every five married men admit that they are still masturbating. The frequency with which this group masturbates is depicted in Figure 8.10. Most (82 percent) do it between one and five times a month. This is, on the average, about once a week.

If my clinical experience is any guide, this means that the average man is alternatively masturbating between every second and third intercourse.

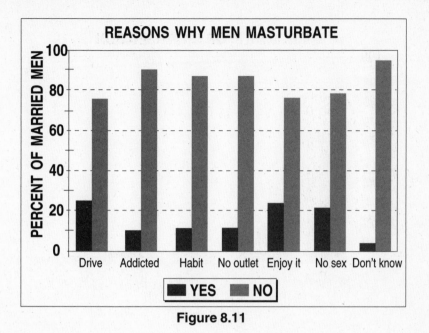

Figure 8.11

I suspect that the strongest reason for this is that his wife isn't ready for sex.

About 10 percent reported an average of between five and ten times per month; 6 percent reported more than fifteen times a month. A very small percentage, about 1 percent, report masturbating more than twenty times a month. This group of men most probably do not have regular sex available for various reasons, including illness of the spouse.

More important to me is the question of why married men masturbate. The reasons they give are depicted in Figure 8.11. They were asked to answer yes or no to a variety of reasons. Bear in mind that it is possible to have more than one reason for masturbating.

The most common reason given was "I have a strong sex drive." Around 23 percent of the men answered yes to this reason. Around 22 percent said it was because they merely enjoyed it. The 23 percent who masturbate because they have a strong sex drive do so, presumably, to supplement their normal sexual outlet with their partner. They enjoy it, probably having learned it early and possibly adding further excitement through pornography. A few share their masturbation with their partner.

Around 21 percent reported that they masturbate because they have no sexual outlet. Sex is not available to them. Their partners are either

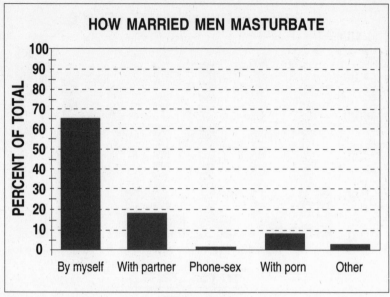

Figure 8.12

not ready or not interested. This means that one in five married males have no sexual outlet other than masturbation. This is the cause of deep personal frustration and dissatisfaction. These marriages desperately need remedial help. They need to find the reason for their sexual dysfunction. Failure here contributes a lot to marital hostility and breakup.

How do married men masturbate? I asked my sample of men to select the settings in which they masturbated, ranging from "by myself" to "with partner," "with phone-sex (900 number)," "with pornography," or "other."

Figure 8.12 presents the results. The majority (66 percent) reported that they masturbated *by themselves*, with no porn or other aids. They may have been stimulated by a movie or by using their imagination, but it is a lonesome experience. Another 19 percent said they did it with their partners either as a mutually shared experience, as a supplement to intercourse, or just in love play. Another 10 percent used porn, and 2 percent called a 900 number for sex-talk.

How do married men feel about their masturbation? I asked them plain and simple, giving them four choices: guilty, shameful, abnormal, or healthy. I suppose I could have added a few more but these seemed to cover all the bases for me.

Figure 8.13 gives the results. Almost all (97 percent) said they did not feel guilty. Only 2 percent said that it was shameful, and 8 percent that it

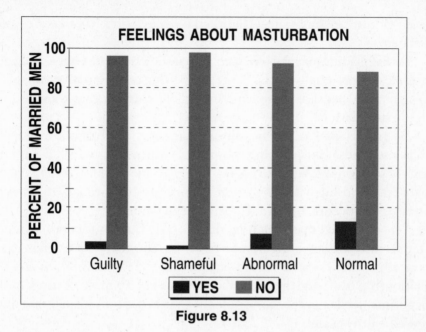

Figure 8.13

was abnormal. But on the other hand, only 13 percent said they felt normal about their masturbation. So what does this mean? Either they genuinely don't know how they feel or they have a lot of ambivalence about their feelings. On the one hand, 97 percent said they don't feel guilty, but only 13 percent said it felt normal.

I believe that what these men really feel about their masturbation is that it is an unfortunate necessity. They would prefer, or at least most of them would, to have a more satisfactory sexual relationship and readily available sexual partner. Since most men masturbate because their partner is not available, ready or interested, they turn to masturbation as a second-best option. While they don't feel guilty about it, as such, they also don't feel good about what they are doing. It is the least of many evils. Gone are the days when men agonized over their masturbation.

Is Masturbation Helpful to a Marriage?

Some of the men who masturbate would probably continue to do so no matter how much sex was available to them. They masturbate because they are hooked on it. Often it accompanies the use of pornography in an obsessive-compulsive disorder. This is becoming a serious sexual problem in our culture and now affects between 6 percent and 10 percent of married men.

As I explained in chapter 3, such sexual addictions are established early in adolescence, usually in the context of strong condemnation or taboos. It is precisely because these experiences are naughty that they become highly stimulating.

Such obsessions are not healthy for marriages. The husband eventually finds intercourse less satisfying. The use of fantasy transports him into the arms of someone else or into his favorite porn movie. He doesn't give his sexual relationship with his partner the priority and intimacy it deserves. There is no incentive to build a better sexual bond.

I have treated many such marriages. The husband spends so much time secretly masturbating that he never has the energy or interest to romance his wife. Because she is not romanced she loses interest, and the relationship cools and dies. The secretiveness of his masturbating, in the meantime, feeds the taboo excitement that keeps him sexually isolated. Not a healthy cycle!

The solution? Wherever possible, and preferably under the direction of a therapist, bring the behavior into the open so it can be a shared experience with the wife. Or to put it bluntly, if you can't stop it, then at least make it a shared experience.

In order to break a sexual obsessive-compulsive disorder, it is vital that there be total honesty and openness. This takes away the guilt component and robs the behavior of some of its unique pleasure. The male won't enjoy it so much, but that is part of the design for healing. Ultimately, the couple can begin to work on restoring some sexual pleasure to their own relationship.

What about the normal husband? He prefers sex over masturbation, has no particular affinity for masturbation and/or pornography, but has a need for sexual relief. Either his wife is not available or she is not interested in sex. I would say that there are three conditions under which masturbation is clearly wrong or destructive:

1. *When it is used to avoid sexual intimacy or to punish a partner by satisfying oneself.* Does this happen? Often. A husband who is angry takes care of himself by self-stimulation and avoids intimacy with his wife as long as possible, hoping she

will "suffer" and be good to him next time. Not only is this psychologically sick, it is downright immoral!

2. *When it is used to fulfill an addictive urge.* Here, as with other addictions, masturbation is used as an emotional anesthesia to numb pain or avoid reality. Some men drink alcohol; others use masturbation. There is little difference, really, in the underlying dynamics.

3. *When it is used to foster lust or a desire for others.* I believe there is something intrinsically immoral about masturbating to fantasies that involve other men's wives or, for that matter, single women. What right does any man have to take my wife in fantasy? What right do I have to take yours?

I do not believe that masturbation itself is morally wrong or, to use the language of the circles I move in, *sinful.* The biblical references most commonly cited as condemning masturbation are often taken out of context or are cited by those who have other agendas. There are many opposing points of view and I want to respect the rights of all. However, the outright and unequivocal condemnation of masturbation without regard to the circumstances causes more problems than it solves. The secretiveness and privateness of masturbation will always remain, in my opinion, its most damaging aspect. And the more we condemn it, the more we keep it secret and private.

I'm all for openness, so let's get masturbation out of the closet. The majority of good men masturbate, though not always for healthy reasons. Teenagers are going to masturbate whether we like it or not. But here is the bottom line: *Solo sex is not a healthy substitute for real sex.*

Mastering Lust

Around 59 percent of my sample of good married men said they find it sexually stimulating to fantasize about having sex with someone other than their wife. A friend recently added, "and the rest are probably lying!" Perhaps not. But even at 59 percent that's a lot of men.

A married minister wrote to me recently and said he has struggled with the problem of lust as far back as he can remember. He has prayed about it, searched the Scriptures about it, read numerous books, and even planned programs to teach sexual abstinence, penance, and mortification. But nothing has helped him. The best sublimation he has ever achieved lasted three days!

This pastor is not alone in his struggle. This thing called lust haunts and tantalizes men beyond words. Partly it is because they are good men that they struggle with it—if they weren't, why would they care?

Not every man who feels sexually aroused or stimulated by another woman is being lustful. Many men just plain notice beauty, and their hormones do their natural thing. There's no point in condemning nature or yourself for having a normal body, good eyesight, and impeccable taste. Some of the most moral men I know are the greatest appreciators of beauty. It's what you do with this arousal that determines whether or not you are being lustful.

The term *lust* implies an overwhelming desire that overtakes you. It is lust, not because it comes and then goes quickly, but because it persists and causes you to long for sexual satisfaction from the one who is stimulating you. Lust means you're obsessing. Lust means you cannot get your mind off of it. Lust means you crave what you can't have. Jesus said "whosoever looketh on a woman to lust after her" is the one who is committing adultery (Matt. 5:28).

The easiest way to break the habit of lust, if it really is lust (and you are the best judge of this) is, first of all, to stop feeling guilty over every twinge of excitement. Accountability to someone else is a great protection. If it is appropriate to your relationship, tell your partner (in a respectful way) when someone you see is attractive. This can help remove your guilt as well as keep you accountable for your roving eyes!

Furthermore, you must discipline your thinking. This is helpful not only in the realm of sexuality but in other areas of your life as well. Men are at high risk for accusations of harassment if they stare uncontrollably. And generally, these are men who have no control over their thinking. Lust occurs without their awareness. They are slaves to desire because they are slaves to a particular style of thinking. How can we discipline our thought-life so as not to fuel the fire of lust?

Realize that lust is a serious problem. Not only is it important for women to feel safe and not be the target of every man's fantasies, but women also need to be viewed other than just as sexual objects. But it's important to us, too. The effect of uncontrolled sexual preoccupation is damaging to our sexual integrity.

Dirty thinking is a habit. All habits are learned and can be unlearned. And like other bad habits, lust is best dealt with by abstaining. To do this you have to catch yourself when you engage in sexual thinking. Set your watch to beep every hour. If you catch yourself dwelling on some sexual fantasy, switch your thinking to something else. Choose what you think about and choose wholesome thoughts. Only in severe cases of obsessional thinking do you lose the ability to choose what you think. And there is treatment available for obsessional thinking, so even that is no excuse. Some men find relief through spiritual resources or prayer. But the habit *must* be changed.

Maintaining Fidelity

"Marriage is all very well; but it isn't romance," wrote George Bernard Shaw in 1916. He may be accurately describing some marriages, but they don't have to be that way. Having worked with many men who avoid marriage, I haven't yet found a man who has been the better for staying single for the wrong reasons.

Marriage is still our last best chance for growing up. It helps to build a happy, contented, and intimate closeness. It is better than therapy. Happily married people of both sexes are among the healthiest in our society.

How to stay married and still be happy is a great challenge. I've done so for thirty-nine years and think I have some answers, but they must wait for another book. Meanwhile, I'd say that one of the key factors in staying happy is to remain committed to one partner. We call it *marital fidelity*.

Confining sex exclusively to one's partner is the *only* way to build a stable, long-lasting, and happy marriage. And choosing to restrict one's sexual focus to one lifelong partner is a basic factor in character building. The quality of person you are is defined by this. It's all a matter of self-discipline. So the apostle Paul could write, "That each one of you should know how to possess [control, manage] his own body (in purity, separated from things profane, and) in consecration and honor" (1 Thess. 4:4 AMP).

Self-control is a key ingredient in all sexual expression. Without self-control not only does society disintegrate, but a person becomes unpredictable and dangerous.

Now in trying to provide guidelines for sexual control, my intention throughout this book has not been to appeal to religious or moral principles, even though I adhere to them. I have stuck with good, old-fashioned common sense.

So let me emphasize here, with regard to the need for marital fidelity, that we all have our price. By this I mean that every one of us, males in particular, have someone of the opposite sex out there other than our wives who is our dream come true—good men, moral men, and religious men not excluded.

For reasons I won't elaborate on here, these women are so appealing to us and are so able to attract us that we would sell our souls, abandon our families, and throw away everything we stand for to be with such a person. In a nutshell, none of us, no matter how moral, is beyond temptation to be unfaithful. If you think you are, "take heed lest you fall."

Am I exaggerating? Aren't there some of us so staid, so moral, so strong-willed, so upright that we would never fall? I don't think so, and I am being thoroughly biblical here. Too often I have watched the most upright, moral, highly committed pastors throw away everything they stand for just to be with the woman of their dreams. Sometimes it's a secretary. Sometimes a parishioner. But they have their price.

Don't think it won't happen to you. And if you ever see your price and you value your family and what you stand for, run away as fast as your legs can carry you. Running away is always the best antidote for temptation! We all have the seeds of unfaithfulness within us, ready to take root at the slightest opportunity.

Who is at risk? There are certain men at greater risk than others. For instance, those at greater risk have some or all of the following characteristics:

- *An innocent outlook.* They are naive about their own vulnerabilities.

- *A high, but rigid, standard of morals.* Rigidity of morals often bespeaks a man whose defenses are brittle and easily broken down. Those who behave as if they are invulnerable are often the most vulnerable.

- *Too many unmet needs.* Men who have never been deeply loved either in childhood or adulthood are more likely to seek out someone to meet these needs. Men who are hungry for affirmation or attention often get unwittingly caught up in affairs.

- ***Too much failure and stress.*** Midlife failure is a common trigger for infidelity. The male reaches out for sexual fulfillment to comfort the pain that a sense of failure brings.

- ***Too much guilt.*** Guilt proneness, rather than being a protection, is often a hazard to fidelity just as it is to obsessiveness. More often than not, it exaggerates the pleasure of an affair.

Marital infidelity is not so much the result of a failure of morality as it is the pressure of psychological or circumstantial factors. When a marriage lacks intimacy, is devoid of mature love, and where there is an avoidance or unwillingness to communicate, you have all the ingredients for an affair. All it takes is a wrong turn down a different street on your way to work and you may meet someone you can idealize. You've met your price. And you'll pay for it out of everything you hold dear!

Another point: most men carry over from their adolescent years the idea that good sex is essentially dirty. Some choose to move *down* the social scale to satisfy their urges. Sometimes this even means going to a prostitute. When highly moral men fall, many times they fall all the way to the gutter. Check out our fallen TV evangelists for proof of this.

This brings me to my final point. Earlier in this chapter I quoted from Paul Tournier's book, *To Understand Each Other.* He states that men clam up because many women make their husbands feel misunderstood, condemned, and even despised about their real inner sexual feelings and temptations. Men withdraw into themselves, form a shell of silence, and stop trying even to communicate superficial feelings about their sexual attractions to other women.

Tournier believes, and I fully support him here, that it is this "veil of silence that may well jeopardize their marriage far more than his sex drive." This is a jewel of insight. The inability to talk about intimate feelings opens the door for sexual infidelity. Ultimately, there is no excuse for any man who has an affair. But everything possible should be done to keep communications open. Tournier makes this brilliant statement:

> The best protection against sexual temptations is to be able to speak honestly of them and to find, in the wife's understanding, without any trace of complicity whatsoever, effective and affective help needed to overcome them.[4]

My wife and I have followed this advice for many years to our great benefit. So work at building an open, honest communication about your sexual feelings. When a man can truly be at one with an understanding partner, becoming normal in his sexuality can be a lot easier.

WHAT TO DO WHEN YOU FIND YOURSELF SEXUALLY ATTRACTED TO ANOTHER WOMAN

1. Avoid being alone with her. Ensure that your spouse is with you whenever you must be with this person.

2. Stop fantasizing about being with her romantically or sexually.

3. Don't open Pandora's box by telling her that you are attracted to her. It will only complicate matters more. She may turn around and accuse you of harassment.

4. Share your feelings of attraction with a close friend who can hold you accountable.

5. Take responsibility for all your actions. You are not to blame for your feelings, but you are responsible for the actions that follow your feelings.

6. Try to look at the whole picture. A moment of passion can lead to a lifetime of regret and hurt.

9

Men, Sex, and the Workplace

How do you spell trouble? Take a man whose sex drive is quite normal and place him in a work setting where he is in close contact with women. Raise the stakes by having the women dress provocatively, or have two or three of them on the lookout for a life partner. Make it even more explosive by adding social activities where alcohol flows freely. The result is always the same—sex in the workplace.

What amazes me is not how often sex occurs in the workplace. I'm astonished that it doesn't occur more often, given the many risk factors associated with the workplace! I'm not referring to sexual harassment, but consentual sex—premarital and extramarital. The average man spends more hours per day with his coworkers than with his wife, thus rendering the average office, factory, or job site a major hazard for the sexual male.

And then there is sexual harassment, the scourge of workplace sexuality. We will never eliminate sexual harassment until we eliminate workplace sex. You'll always have the one if you have the other.

Sex and the Workplace

How common is sex in the workplace? *The Janus Report* provides some fairly reliable estimates. It differs from region to region. In the West and Northeast 38 percent and 36 percent of both sexes admitted to having had a sexual experience once or twice on the job. The remaining 62 percent said they have never had a sexual encounter at work. In the Midwest and South, between 22 percent and 24 percent admitted to having had a sexual experience while on the job.

Roughly speaking, then, we can assume that between a quarter and third of both men and women have engaged in workplace sex. Most have only done it once or twice. Only 2 percent to 4 percent have done it often.

Why are the figures higher in the West and Northeast? This is where many of the major cities are located. In large cities people have to travel farther to work, are away from home longer, and experience greater stress and less personal support than in small towns. Also, we know that moral values tend to be diminished in large cities.

But from their interview with large numbers of men, the Januses concluded that workplace sex is not so much a consequence of urban settings as it is of the abuse of power and control. The man's sexual pleasure might very well be experienced by women as sexual harassment.[1]

The Januses found that between one-third and one-half of the women reported sexual harassment on the job. I am sure there are many instances where women were eager and willing participants in workplace encounters. Genuine two-sided affairs between consenting adults happen all the time. But quite often the seduction is one-sided, with a man taking advantage of some weakness on the woman's side. Furthermore, some exploitative men promise a long-term relationship when in fact they have no such intention. Their promises are designed to help their seductions.

Unfortunately, in today's dating climate it is quite common for women to believe that the only way to catch a man is to have sex with him. Or to put it another way, "unless you have sex with your date you will never see him again." What a lie! If a man can get milk for nothing, why would he want to buy a cow?

Women who are taken advantage of in this way have every right to feel used, even abused. While in the strictest legal sense it may not constitute harassment, it is exploitation of a woman's vulnerability, and that is just as despicable. I strongly believe that the point of control in all sexual matters is with the man, not the woman. This means that we have a lot of work to do in educating young males about the true nature of their sexuality. They must learn to see women as colleagues, not as sexual objects.

In my sample, 94 percent of the men reported that they worked in close proximity to women. Their contacts ranged from supervising

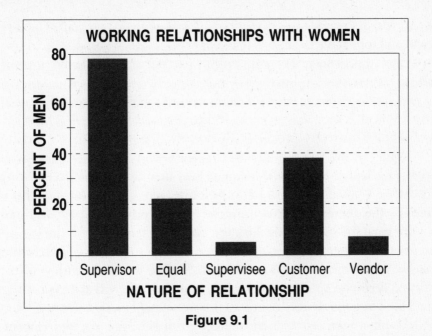

Figure 9.1

women to having them as customers or vendors. Figure 9.1 presents the varieties of contacts experienced.

Most (78 percent) of the men reported that they in some way or other supervised women. Only about 7 percent reported that they were supervised by women, reflective of the male dominance in the work force. Around 39 percent reported that they had women as customers of one sort or another. They could be business customers or women in a parish, presuming the man being surveyed is a clergyman.

Workplace sex does not only occur between coworkers or between a boss and employee. It also occurs between those who deliver a service and the women they serve: salesmen selling cars, technicians repairing telephones, college professors teaching classes, reporters interviewing someone, preachers who go to comfort the sick or divorced. Put men and women together in any work setting and you can get trouble.

Sexual Harassment

Every day, every hour, indeed every minute, a working woman in the United States suffers in some way because of a male's out-of-control sex drive. About fifty thousand sexual harassment lawsuits were filed between 1980 and 1990 in the U.S. Something is seriously wrong.

I can almost hear the male's protests: "But women also harass men. We aren't the only culprits!" True. But I searched my clinical records hard to come up with a case where a man has really suffered serious damage, or any damage, from a woman's sexual harassment. Couldn't find one! Men seldom suffer the way women do, although it does happen.

A man in the Los Angeles area recently won a million-dollar lawsuit against his female boss who threatened him after he had rejected her sexual advances. The man alleged he was sexually harassed almost daily for six years by the company's chief financial officer and director of personnel.[2]

Despite the exceptions, let's use common sense. By far the greatest number of harassment cases occur with men as the initiators. And the message we must send to men is simply this: Women who work with you are at risk and deserve respect and protection from being viewed as sexual objects.

I have refrained from saying "merely as sexual objects," because I don't believe most men see women "merely" in this way. They may respect a woman's talent, affirm her contribution to the organization, and even envy her competence but still look at her through sex-tinted glasses. They undress women in their minds, fantasize about them in their imaginations, and eventually give themselves away with an inadvisable comment. This may be a slip of the tongue, but the tongue is connected to a mind that is bathed in testosterone much of the time.

So my concern here is not with blatant harassment—the kind that makes the papers—but with the subtle, attitudinal distortions that occur in the minds of all ordinary good men. Believe me, even this can be very destructive over the long haul.

Do Good Men Sexually Harass Women?

Do good men sexually harass women at work or in a social situation? Unfortunately they do. I recently talked with a young pastor's wife. In her early thirties, she is very attractive. She never plays up her attractiveness by over (or under) dressing, is quite discreet in her behavior toward men, and always communicates a strong attachment to her husband. You'd think this behavior would communicate a clear and unambiguous message to the males of the church. Not so.

For this young pastor's wife—let's call her Pat—life has become a living hell. A deacon in her church, at least ten years her senior, has become fixated on her. By all accounts, this deacon has a solid marriage, solid kids, and a solid existence. He is honest, moral, and spiritual. He is a really good man, but his sexual feelings are out of control.

His fixation on the pastor's wife has never caused him to do anything that would constitute formal harassment. It is subtle, covert, and hidden, an aggravating presence that Pat feels more than she can prove. In fact, she's often tried to prove to her husband that what she feels is genuine, but he refuses to acknowledge it. Perhaps he's afraid of facing the consequences.

Pat knows without a doubt that this deacon is fixated on her. He stares at her all the time but when she turns her head he quickly turns away. He hangs around and makes excuses to talk to her. When he thinks she's not looking, he glances at her breasts. When she walks away, he stares at her legs. She saw him do this several times by catching his reflection in the large glass window in the church's foyer.

Does this constitute harassment? It certainly does. While he has never even spoken an inappropriate word to her, tried to become a special friend, or ever made any moves, his fixation has caused Pat tension and anxiety.

Pat's husband thinks that maybe she's the one with the crush. "What am I supposed do?" he pleads with her. "Everyone believes the guy is Mr. Upright. I would end up making a fool of myself and you if I challenged him about the way he looks at you."

A man's sexual interest, even if only expressed from a distance, can be a major source of fear in a woman. It can be distressing and even injurious. Sexual harassment can escalate from overfriendliness to excessive staring to inappropriate or frequent touching. It's *all* harassment because it *all* causes discomfort, fear, even repugnance to a woman who doesn't want it.

Gender Harassment in the Workplace

A common idea in feminist circles is that sexual harassment, like rape, is largely an abuse of power and control, perhaps even a form of rage. I would counter that the most common reason men engage in harassing behavior is that their sexual urges are out of control. It may be experienced by women as a form of violence, but for the male it is a drive for sex.

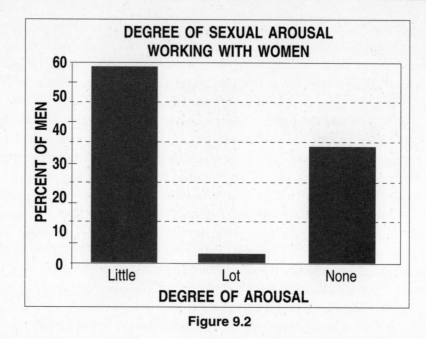

Figure 9.2

There is harassment of women that is gender-based but sexual as such. We call it gender harassment, and it is different from sexual harassment. Unfortunately we don't distinguish between the two clearly enough. Gender-based harassment is often violent, motivated by rage. It might, as with rape, involve a degree of sexuality, but the remark or act is designed to hurt, not excite or satisfy a sexual need. It is raw hostility, and the anger is directed at a woman.

For instance, blue-collar workers have been known to taunt and jeer women who have moved into their masculine sphere of work. These women have been given faulty or dangerous equipment to work with, have been locked in vaults, and even threatened with physical harm.[3] Even male physicians have made life miserable for female doctors intruding into their domain. This is gender harassment, not sexual harassment. My work with men leads me to believe that genuine sexual harassment arises when the male's sex drive is out of control. It may be fostered by a low view of women but is essentially sexual in nature.

Not all men are vindictive fiends trying to take revenge on the opposite sex because they've been abused, rejected, or humiliated by a woman. There are exceptions, but this is not true for most men. For the men I know, the problem is with sexual desire. "Think about sex all the time,"

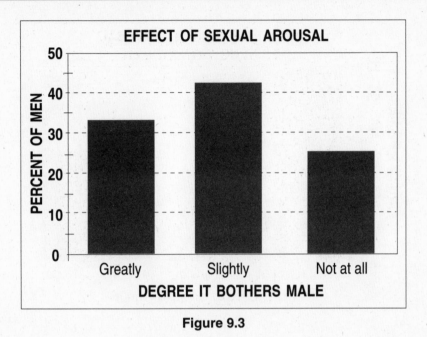

Figure 9.3

their hormones tell them. "Take whatever opportunity you can to get all the sex you can," their programming dictates. It's not right, and it's not pretty—but that's how it is.

Sexual Arousal in the Workplace

How much sexual arousal do men experience in the workplace? I asked my men the question, "Does working around women cause you any sexual arousal?" Options were a little, a lot, or not at all. Figure 9.2 presents the results. Around 59 percent reported a little sexual arousal, meaning that for the majority of men the workplace is somewhat sexually stimulating—not overpowering, but noticeable. Only 36 percent said they felt no sexual arousal at work, and 3 percent reported a lot of sexual arousal. This means that about one male in thirty is having a serious problem with sexual feelings on the job. This doesn't represent a lot of men, but they are there in every office, workshop, or construction site—enough to be a source of sexual harassment.

How is sexual arousal in the workplace experienced? Figure 9.3 presents the results. Just under 42 percent say it bothers them slightly. They

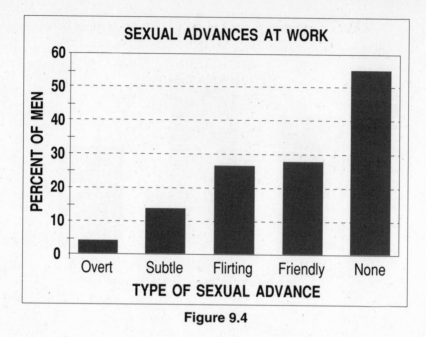

Figure 9.4

notice it, but can put it out of their minds. They don't dwell on it nor do they make anything more of it.

But 32 percent said it bothered them greatly. That makes about one in three men who find their sexual feelings a real interference. Only 25 percent said it didn't bother them at all. So including those men who were slightly or greatly bothered, we can account for 74 percent—three out of every four men—in the workplace.

Workplace sexual arousal, enough to be noticed, is therefore a very common experience in men, even good men, and cannot be minimized as a major source of possible harassment. Being bothered means that it gets your attention. The fact that it bothers you may mean that you can't concentrate on what you should be doing because your arousal is too distracting. It can even mean that it gives you pleasure and that you indulge it deliberately.

Do men receive sexual advances themselves? They are always being accused of being the instigators in sexual activities, but is this always true? I posed this question, "Do you ever encounter any of the following at work?" Options ranged from "overt sexual advances" to "flirtations."

Figure 9.4 presents the results. Just under 5 percent of the men reported that they had received overt sexual advances from female coworkers. One

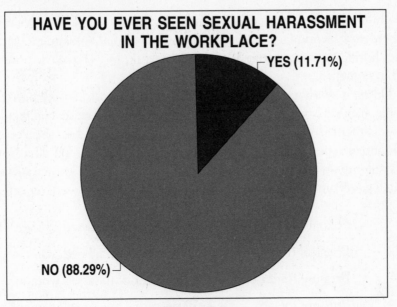

HAVE YOU EVER SEEN SEXUAL HARASSMENT IN THE WORKPLACE?

YES (11.71%)

NO (88.29%)

Figure 9.5

in twenty! That's quite a fair number of men, considering how many there are in the work force. Can we trust men to give a true answer here? After all, men generally have a much narrower definition of sexual harassment and are likely to blame women for instigating the harassment.

I have no reason not to believe these men. They have no reason to be defensive. A few may be engaging in wishful thinking, believing that a woman's friendliness has other motives, but overall, I think it is a fair estimate. It certainly corroborates my clinical experience.

Nearly 14 percent of the men reported subtle sexual advances. Here we probably have a few exaggerators. Their emotional eyesight is myopic; they see sex in everything. But even if we discount a few of these men who are exaggerating or misreading cues we are looking at nearly 20 percent, or one in five men, who have been confronted with what they believe to be an overt or subtle sexual advance from a woman.

Flirtations in the workplace are even more common yet are equally dangerous. Around 28 percent of the men reported flirting on the job. Over-friendliness with a female was reported at a slightly higher rate (29 percent), and probably includes the flirtations category as well. More than half (55 percent) reported never seeing any inappropriate behaviors on the part of either men or women on the job. This is a classic "is the glass half full or half empty?" dilemma. On the one hand we can say that 50 percent of workplaces are free of potential sexual harassment. On the other hand, we can say that 50 percent of workplaces have the potential for harassment.

Do men really notice sexual harassment at work? In my particular sample, nearly 12 percent of the men reported having seen several incidents of harassment in the workplace (see Figure 9.5). How does this compare with actual reports of harassment? It depends, of course, on what sort of harassment you mean. In what is probably the most well known survey of female government employees, the following incidents were reported:

Sexual remarks   33 percent of harassed women

Physical touching   26 percent of harassed women

Pressure for dates   15 percent of harassed women

Pressure for sex   10 percent of harassed women[4]

My sample's report of the 12 percent of the men reporting having seen incidents of harassment refers to workplaces where there was harassment. The above statistics refer to women who were harassed. Since some workplaces are likely to have several women being harassed, to say that 12 percent of the men, each representing a different workplace, have seen sexual harassment seems a reasonably accurate estimate. We can then assume that about one in eight workplaces have some sexual harassment going on.

What do men believe about sexual harassment laws? How fair do men perceive the present laws governing sexual harassment to be? Figure 9.6 presents the results. It is startling that 39 percent of the men I surveyed, who are generally well-educated professional men, reported not knowing anything about what the law says on this matter. Perhaps they are in situations that are so safe that they are not required to know, but I doubt it. These men are walking on the edge of a precipice because ignorance of the law is no excuse.

Are the laws fair? One-third of men believed the laws to be fair to both men and women. They saw no bias against men and believe that women need the protection those laws provide.

But 18 percent of the men (approaching one in five) believed that these laws are fair only to women. They probably would assert that these

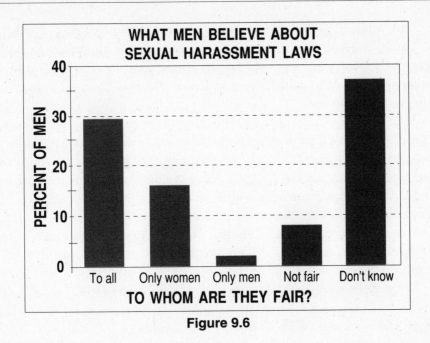

Figure 9.6

laws give women unreasonable power to sue and would also blame women for most of the harassment. There are quite a few men who would like to see us return to the old days when men could assert their sexuality, say what they like, take what they desired, and not concern themselves with the consequences for women. Thank God they are in the minority.

Sexy Dressers on the Job

What I am about to say next won't be popular in some circles. But it needs to be said. Every man would want me to say it, so here goes. The extreme feminist position says that a woman should be able to wear short skirts or see-through blouses if she likes. Men shouldn't notice. "It's not our problem but theirs—don't blame us for a man's sex drive." I can't accept this.

I am not suggesting that women, in general, are in any way responsible for a male's improper sexual response in the workplace. There is never any excuse for harassment. But women must also accept the possibility that when they flaunt their sexuality, men will notice *and will be aroused*.

The solution to sexual harassment in the workplace lies primarily with men, but women need help in understanding male sexuality. Both men and women need to cooperate in a joint venture that will remove harassment from the workplace and sexual violence from all aspects of male/female relations.

Many men feel, rightly or wrongly, that there are women in the workplace playing sexual games. Magazines that cater to the romantic side of a woman's life provide all sorts of advice on how to be seductive and get a man. *Cosmopolitan*, read by a large number of single women, instructs them how to take "indirect initiatives at work to which men unconsciously respond." Initiatives like dropping a pile of papers or a purse, then stooping down to gather them up. "He'll help," they say. "Lean close to him." The advice goes on to say, "If you have good legs, wear a tight, short skirt." "Brush up against somebody in the elevator."[5]

What if the wrong man responds? Do these women really think that *only* the man targeted for the attraction initiative will notice? Men have a right to be concerned about double standards here.

If we really want to eliminate problems with sexuality in the workplace, then something will have to be done about how *some women dress*. Men are human. They have enough problems learning how to control their sex drive as it is without having to work with women who dress skimpily. How much imposed sexual stimulation does a man have to put up with? I believe men have a right to say, "Stop tantalizing me," whether there is a risk of harassment or not.

Bob is genuinely a good man. He loves his wife, loves his kids, and loves his job. He is also a strongly committed Christian in the healthiest way. But some women in his workplace are driving him crazy. He works in a large office as a junior-level executive and relates to a large number of employees, most of whom are female and young.

Most of the women in his office are single. Because he is a nice person and relatively good looking, the women like him a lot. They like to be around him. He is always respectful, understands all about sexual harassment, and has never, ever acted inappropriately. So what's the problem?

Many of these women dress provocatively. Do they have a clue about what effect their dressing has on men? Yes and no. They dress in a certain way to attract male attention and admiration. But do they realize that when a healthy man sees a lot of thigh, tight skirts or low-cut blouses, he has a pretty good chance of becoming aroused and even getting an erection? This happens all the time to healthy men—both bad men and good men.

Bob tries hard not to notice how these women dress. He distracts himself as much as he can. When the provocation is very strong, he takes long walks at lunchtime to work off his arousal. If the office building had cold showers he'd be the cleanest, coldest man in the place.

Recently Bob was conducting a staff meeting. One young lady walked over to show him something, bent forward, and almost everything she possessed above the waist was exposed. She didn't mean anything by it. She wasn't trying to be seductive; in fact, she was totally oblivious to what was happening. Bob nearly freaked out. The arousal was overwhelming. He excused himself on the pretext of making an urgent telephone call and left the meeting.

Is Bob unusual in this respect? Is he atypical? Not at all. Almost every man I know would be affected the same way Bob was. I don't know any mental technique that can stop sexual arousal in the normal male when breasts are displayed in such a way. I know physicians who can examine a nude breast and feel no response, but they can become extremely excited by a low-cut dress. Oh, the mysteries of male sexuality. Oh, the hazards it creates on the job.

Seeing a lot of the female body at the beach may not be very stimulating. But a dress that inadvertently creeps up can drive a man to distraction. This is one of the strange aspects of sexual stimulation, as every male will confess. Total nudity is not as stimulating as partial nudity. *Intrigue* plays a crucial role in visual stimulation, and inadvertent exposure is more stimulating then deliberate exposure.

How can we teach these facts to women?

But back to Bob. With my encouragement he took up the issue of how women dressed at work with upper management. At first he didn't get a lot of support. Some thought he was being a fuddy-duddy and too old-fashioned. The truth is, most of the men who worked with him liked what they saw. They thrived on their daily dose of stimulation, boasting that their firm had a reputation for hiring pretty women. They used it even as a recruiting incentive for top executives. This firm's upper management was extremely sexist.

When allegations of sexual harassment began to surface, however, management soon sat up and paid attention. Pressure was applied for

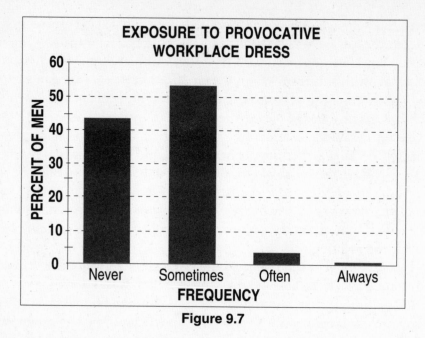

Figure 9.7

dress to be more modest. I realize this is a delicate matter. Conflicting interests are at stake. Why should women have to consider how they dress, just because men can't control their sexual hormones?

To find out how often men experienced this sort of provocation—short skirts, low-cut blouses, tight clothes, and the like—I asked my sample for their response. Figure 9.7 gives the results.

Around 42 percent of the men reported that they are never exposed to provocative dress by women. But 53 percent said they were exposed sometimes and only 4 percent said they were exposed often. A very small percentage, just under 1 percent, said they were always exposed to sexually provocative dress. About 58 percent of the men, then, are sometimes or often exposed to dress that sexually provokes them.

How do they experience this exposure? Figure 9.8 tells the story quite clearly. One in three males (33 percent), reported that provocative dress causes them sexual arousal. For some men this means an erection. It will almost certainly mean accelerated heartbeat and sexual excitement.

Only 3.9 percent of the men reported that their experience of provocative dress was enjoyable. It seems to me that enjoying is a precursor to arousal. Clearly, being aroused on the job is neither good for the job or for the women who work there.

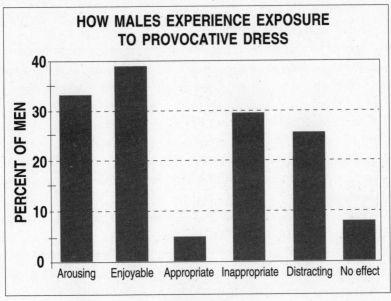

Figure 9.8

Around 29 percent of the men reported that the reaction that provocative dress caused them was inappropriate. Whether they were aroused or just enjoyed it, they knew that what they were feeling was not appropriate. Good for them. It violated either their own standards or the rights of the woman involved. One out of four (25 percent) of the men reported that when they are exposed to provocative dress it distracts them from their work. This is probably the same group who found their reactions to be inappropriate. Only 8 percent said it had no effect and didn't bother them at all.

Provocative dress is not neutral. It does have a distracting effect on men. To experience, even occasionally, sexual arousal toward a woman because of the way she dresses is bound to set the stage for some sort of an inappropriate response, the stuff of which much sexual harassment is made.

How, Then, Should Men Behave?

There is no doubt that we need a revolution in the way men think about women. We need to create a generation or two of males who are in control of their sexual responsiveness. Once they are able to view all women, no matter how they dress, as nonsexual objects, we will be able to declare the workplace safe for women.

Will we ever be able to achieve such a Utopia? Probably not. This means that business owners, departmental heads, and CEOs need to take some responsibility, if not all of it, for seeing that the workplace is safe *for both sexes*. Men may not be at any great risk for harassment on the job, but they deserve protection from an overtly sexually stimulating environment.

A lot of men won't complain when a woman dresses skimpily or flaunts her sexual attractiveness. They like it. They relish it. They occasionally slip to the restroom to secretly masturbate, fantasizing about whatever has turned them on.

Men must own their responsibility. Women are at work to earn a living, not to provide distraction from unrewarding or monotonous chores. Men should endeavor to retrain their thinking and change their attitudes about women. I know it's hard, but they should respect a woman's right to privacy. This means looking away when a voluptuous supervisor has to bend over to pick up a dropped file. It means averting the eyes when an already-short dress creeps up a few extra inches. Eyes can also be intrusive, not just hands. Just looking can be as harassing as any suggestive remark when it is uninvited and unwanted.

Those in charge must take ultimate responsibility for the protection of all workers. In considering the effects of an intrusive sexuality, they need to consider both *risk* and *protective* factors.

Risk factors include harboring in the work force men who are known to be harassers, who demonstrate that they cannot contain their sexual interests. Some men are persistent seducers. They live for conquering women, and the more resistant a woman appears, the more excited they become about the chase. Even if the victims of such seduction never complain, such men pose a significant risk to others. A wise boss will have them removed.

There are also women who pose a significant risk factor. They may not be as common as out-of-control men, but they are there. They caricature their femininity and constantly seek male attention. Innocent, good men are sometimes deceived by the lure of such women. They are lively, flirtatious, but immature. They crave novelty, stimulation, and excitement and quickly become bored with normal routine. Most of all they communicate to men an appealing sexual abandonment, giving off vibes that say, "I'll do anything. Nothing you can imagine is outside my ability."

Men fall for it. Good men. Smart men. Married men. Every church has one of these women, so pastors beware. Most workplaces have a few, so workers be careful. Why? Because when thwarted, these women turn vicious. They are the "fatal attraction" types. If you get involved then withdraw, these women will threaten suicide, damage your car, and destroy your family.

Protective factors include on-the-job training for both sexes about the hazards of workplace sex, AIDS, and provocative dress. Companies and organizations can limit social activities, setting up parties, picnics, and other events so that they include spouses and families. Naturally, they also are responsible for making the laws of sexual harassment clear and understood by every employee.

Prevention is better than cure, especially when it comes to sex in the workplace.

Violence Against Women

No matter where the abuse takes place, our society has failed to grasp the scope or seriousness of violence against women. Rape, spouse abuse, and the victimization of women as sexual objects is epidemic. Much of this violence, I believe, has sexual roots. Husbands beat their wives because they don't give them sex. Teenagers date-rape because they can't control their sex drive. Men harass women in the workplace either because they view all women as sexual objects or because they are trying to get a sense of sexual domination or revenge.

To solve these problems, attention has to be given to how male sexuality is formed and distorted. Legislation is important, but far more important is our urgent need to address what is happening to our boys as they develop their sexuality. We do too little to prepare them for the sexual lion's den that awaits them on the job.

Sexuality can never be confined just to the bedroom. It permeates all social settings and will certainly never be controlled by legalism. Like it or not, men carry it with them all the time. But sexuality can be controlled. And that control can best be achieved by developing, at the deepest level, the right attitudes and beliefs, both about sex in general and women in particular.

QUIZ FOR WOMEN

Do you dress to please or dress to tease?

1. Do you wear tight skirts or dresses around certain men or at certain meetings?

2. Do you wear low-cut tops or allow your cleavage to show?

3. Do you wear see-through blouses, even though you have no slip underneath?

4. Do you bend down, sit, or walk in a manner that causes a man to notice you in a sexual way?

Please remember . . . some men are aroused by what their imagination does with what they see, so be respectful and aware. Before leaving for the office, check your outfit. Are you contributing to male sexual arousal? Hopefully, the women who work around your boyfriend or your present or future husband will be equally respectful.

10

Religion and Sex

"I must confess I find the relationship between religion and sex to be confusing." These are not the words of an atheist or antireligious zealot, but those of a sincere pastor. He continues:

> I don't have problems with affirming the ideas of no sex before marriage or marital fidelity. These seem quite reasonable to me. What I have problems with is trying to harmonize my Christian beliefs with such issues as oral sex, masturbation after marriage, anal sex, and whatever else gives a couple pleasure. These are difficult areas for me, not only personally, but in the counseling work I do. I just don't know what is right or wrong. I suppose that if I were not religious, these issues would not bother me at all.

This pastor's dilemma is a very common one in conservative Christian circles. I suspect that it is a problem for certain other religious groups as well. The relationship between religion, with its moral demands, and sex, with its tendency to test the appropriate boundaries of morality, has never been a harmonious one. Much confusion, misinformation, and conflict exist throughout Protestant, Catholic, and even Jewish religious groups.

Sex and religion seem to be working against each other. Opponents of religion often try to prove two opposing ideas: either that to be religious, even to the slightest extent, inhibits our sexuality or that religion turns us into repressed sexual perverts or raving sexual maniacs. People of faith can't win.

A major component in religion's impact on sexuality involves the mechanism of guilt. To some extent, all religions use guilt to enforce moral codes. People are taught self-control by being made to feel bad whenever they do something wrong. Is this all bad? I don't think so. However, as I have said before, it is important to differentiate healthy guilt from neurotic or false guilt. My remarks here are primarily directed at Christianity because that is my faith. I don't believe there is anything wrong with Christianity. However, certain practices within the Christian culture can lead to distortions of guilt, and that is my primary concern here.

We have either religion or the law to offer behavioral control. Since we can't make a law for every behavior, we depend heavily on religion, especially its moral codes. Not surprisingly, religion messes up our sexuality occasionally because religion is the only system left that cares about our deepest well-being. When sex gets out of control, sexuality ends up being in conflict with our faith.

Religion's Relationship with Sex

Religion and sex have had a long relationship together. Sometimes it has been a good relationship, sometimes destructive. For many centuries, religion was a primary force regulating sexual practices. Sex was also a part of some religious systems. Even today we occasionally encounter a religious cult that tries to include uninhibited sexual expression as a part of its worship. Recently, one group's high priestess (in California, of course) initiated all new male members with sex. The courts found it was a glorified form of prostitution.

Sometimes religion and sex are constructively linked. In ancient India, religious rules helped keep men chaste and wives faithful. Women were forbidden to worship with men or to attend social functions while their husbands were away. Privacy, isolation, and privileged position were enjoined on women. Out of this came the *Kama Sutra*, a sexual guide so complete that it lists seven different ways of kissing, eight varieties of touch, and eight playful bites.

In this religious system, sex was seen to be a pleasurable activity as much for the woman as for the man and one from which everyone could derive the richest experiences of life. Religious feelings and sexuality at their highest level, without perversity, were seen to be a deeply religious experience.

Sex and religion are both essential components of human existence. The first sexual act recorded in the Bible appears in Genesis 4:1 where we are told that "Adam *knew* Eve his wife," (emphasis is mine.) Humans, like all animals, have a sexual side, but they also have a religious need. Both sex and religion can provide ecstatic experiences, so it is not surprising that they have become linked in human history.

Both Jewish and Christian religious views embrace sexuality as a gift from God and see it as a part of God's intention for creation. Furthermore, this God-given sexuality includes sexual intercourse.[1] Not only is intercourse a spiritual symbol of "becoming one" but this idea is used throughout Scripture to symbolize the relationship of God to persons.

Traditional Jewish and Christian teaching may see intercourse as a God-given blessing, but they differ in what they teach about sexual pleasure. A major issue that has religious origins is whether sex is *just for procreation or whether it is also for pleasure.*

The Jewish and Catholic religions have traditionally taught that the only purpose for sex is reproduction. Anything outside of this purpose, broadly speaking of course, is sin. This doesn't mean you can't enjoy sex. It just means that there is a limit on what you can do to prevent reproduction in your drive for pleasure.

Protestants, however, are not so dogmatic. While beliefs vary greatly, even the most fundamentalist Christian group accepts that sexual pleasure, for its own sake, is a gift from God. John Calvin taught that it was, so much of the reformed tradition in mainstream Christianity has no problem with this. They don't object to contraception even though they oppose abortion. This is because they see a big difference between *preventing* pregnancy and *terminating* it.

Protestants believe that sex just for pleasure is okay. We have sex to reproduce, but we also have sex for the pleasure it gives those in love. I am emphasizing this point here because there are a lot of deeply religious people who still feel extremely guilty about the pleasure they derive from sex. I know because I encounter them often.

There is no basis for this guilt in Protestant Christian teaching. If you want to know about the real pleasures of sex, read the Song of Solomon in the Bible. It will knock your socks off! I suspect that if some of the really pious people I know were to encounter the Song of Solomon for the first time in adulthood and did not know it was from the Bible, they'd label it as pornographic. They would gather up all the copies they could get their hands on and burn them! Not only is it beautiful poetry, but it extols the deepest joys sex can provide. And it is God-given. Couples would do themselves a lot of good if they read it together on a regular basis to get a spiritual sense of what the sensuality of sex is all about.

Does Religion Always Have a Negative Influence?

Because religious beliefs and practices have always been the primary forces in helping humans regulate their sexuality, we need to ask the question, Is its influence always positive? Are there not times when it is damaging? Let me say at the outset that religious influences, and here I specifically mean Christian religious beliefs, can definitely have a negative influence on sexuality. This happens if beliefs are taught in the wrong context or are enforced in the wrong way.

However, religious beliefs of the good and sound variety have taken the rap unfairly for sex that has gone bad in our Christian subculture. Too often, when someone has ended up as a sexual addict or pervert, critics of religion have blamed Christian parents or the church for the problem. These individuals do not want to take the responsibility for their lives.

One young man I know, not a homosexual, tragically died of AIDS in his late twenties. He blamed his family. "If my parents hadn't been so hung up on religion, I wouldn't have screwed around as much as I did, and I wouldn't have caught AIDS," he complained to me bitterly.

I knew his parents, so I told him bluntly, "Stop blaming your parents. You made certain choices and now you're reaping the consequences."

What Do Researchers Say about Religion and Sex?

Apart from my own surveys, I know of only one other study that makes a serious attempt to look at how religious factors influence sexuality in our modern world. It will serve as an example of how easy it is to misread statistics and blame religion unfairly. I refer to the section in *The Janus Report* that deals with religion and sex.

Despite their own warning that "one must be cautious of erroneous interpretations" because of the wide differences among religions, the authors clearly overstep the mark of cautious interpretation several times.[2] *The Janus Report,* in rather dramatic fashion, states in an opening sidebar at the beginning of its chapter on religion and sex that 30 percent of those who considered themselves to be very religious have had extramarital sexual relations at least once and that 70 percent had had premarital sexual experiences.[3]

Newsweek, picking up on this report, goes on to state that "very religious people actually cheat on their spouses more than plain old religious people."[4] Other supposedly interesting statistics that "give liberals and nonreligious persons fodder for their battles against conservatives" (which is how *Newsweek* reported these findings) include the following:

- Only 51 percent of Protestants and 16 percent of Jewish believers say that their sexual practices are in harmony with their religion. *Implication:* Religious people are hypocrites.

- Only 63 percent of Protestants, less than the 77 percent of nonreligious people, say that masturbation is a natural part of life and continues in marriage. *Implication:* Religious people have sexual hang-ups.

- Around 20 percent of very religious people, versus 10 percent of nonreligious people, say that pain and pleasure really go together in sex. *Implication:* The more religious you are, the more you are likely to be into kinky sex. In fact, the Januses go so far as to say that "the religious actually outstrip the general population in sexual practices that may be considered unconventional."[5]

- Religious and very religious people fantasize about sex (18 percent and 25 percent) more than expected. *Implication:* Religious people are more likely to want to have illicit sex.

- Around 19 percent of very religious men versus 13 percent of nonreligious men, have had full sexual relations by the age of fourteen. *Implication:* The more religious you are, the more likely you'll have early teenage sex.

I could go on, but there is one closing comment worthy of attention. It is made without justification by the authors of *The Janus Report*. It is this: "Religious people have difficulty enjoying their sex lives." Really? If this means that very religious people don't engage in the same kinky or way-out sexual practices of nonreligious people, then it is probably true. But "difficulty enjoying their sex lives"? There is not a shred of evidence for this statement. Not in their own report and not in my work with many very religious men nor in my study.

Response to The Janus Report

As far as the percentages reported by the Januses are concerned, I take no issue. Facts are facts. However, their *interpretation* of the facts is quite another matter. Let me respond briefly to each of their claims:

1. *Are very religious people more likely to have extramarital sexual relations than less religious people?* The difficulty with this type of research lies in how you define *religious*. One needs to know something about the psychology of religion. For instance, one approach in studying religious variables is to separate the two major types of religious people: those who are "extrinsically" religious and those who are "intrinsically" so.

   Extrinsically religious people have an external religion. They go to church. They go to mass. They say their prayers, and they may even consider themselves to be very religious. But little of it impacts them deep within, at a very personal level.

   Intrinsically religious people experience their religion as a deeply personal, subjective thing. They feel it. They are worshiping whether they are in a church or not.

   When we study religious people and make comparisons, we need to reckon with these differences. Both *very* religious and *slightly* religious people can be either extrinsically or intrinsically religious. Some people say they are very religious simply because they go to church regularly, keep the Sabbath, or say their prayers. They may not have any inner sense of deep spirituality or piety.

A second point is this: A person may be deeply religious now but have had a very loose sexual life before conversion. There is no connection between past extramarital affairs and present religious practices. A lot of very religious people I know will admit to a pretty raunchy sexual past. But now they are different.

So these categories are meaningless unless probed further. By their own statistics, however, the Januses are in effect saying that you're better off being very religious here than nonreligious. I'll accept this.

2. *Are very religious people (Jews or Christians) more likely to be hypocritical about their religious/sexual connections? The Janus Report* suggests that in very religious people there is greater conflict between what they do and what they believe. They also conclude that just because "a person places great emphasis on the importance of his or her religious beliefs does not mean that, in that person's private life, there is no deviation."[6]

What are the facts? Around 81 percent of very religious people versus only 26 percent of slightly religious people said "that it is important that my sex practices be in harmony with my religion." They are not saying that their behavior isn't in harmony, just that it is *important* that it be in harmony. This is a statement of intent. This simply means that religious people place great importance "on avoiding contradictions between beliefs and practices in the area of sex."[7]

Is this not what one would expect? Perhaps a religious man's behavior doesn't quite match up to his beliefs. Chances are they won't always because he is only human. Isn't it better for him to have high standards he can't quite meet rather than low standards that don't amount to a hill of beans?

3. *Do religious people have more hang-ups than nonreligious people?* By and large, *The Janus Report* as well as my own study shows that Protestants, including conservatives, now accept masturbation provided it is not obsessive or out of control. Both mental health professionals (including Christians) and medical people see it as a natural part of growing up that may continue on in marriage. In an earlier chapter I advocated that masturbation in married men should, as far as possible, be a shared experience with one's partner. Teenage boys should be taught to limit their self-exploration and experimentation.

   The Januses report that 63 percent of Protestants, compared to 77 percent of nonreligious people, now accept masturbation as normal and healthy. The lower acceptance rate for Protestants is most likely due to some who believe that uncontrolled masturbation is not desirable. Only religious people, it seems, have such concerns or struggle with these issues.

4. *Are religious people more likely than the general population to do something unnatural or kinky? The Janus Report* states that 20 percent of very religious people say that "pain and pleasure often go together" in sex. Only 10 percent of nonreligious people say this.[8]

   In saying that pain and pleasure often go together in sex, very religious people are not admitting that they engage in sadomasochistic behavior. If anything, these religious people are demonstrating their sensitivity to how sex can be abusive in our broken world. Many devout Christian people I know are much more aware of how sex can be destructive than their non-Christian counterparts. If I had answered this question I would certainly have agreed that pain and sex go together. I have seen too many sexual-abuse cases not to answer otherwise. But please don't call me a sadomasochist!

5. *Are religious people more likely to want to have sex with someone other than their wives?* This suggestion comes from the statistic that very religious people (28 percent) fantasize about sex

a great deal, at least more than expected. And since mental sex usually involves a person other than one's partner, these religious people must also want to do this in reality.

I know that very religious men fantasize about having sex with other women. I've already reported on this in an earlier chapter. But if very religious men do this (18 percent) then nonreligious men do it even more (26 percent). My point is that religious men fantasize about sex less than nonreligious men.

6. *Are you more likely to have sex before age fourteen if you are religious than if you are not?* What is implied by this suggestion is that a highly restrictive upbringing is likely to cause young people to act sexually. I'll have more to say about this later when I present the results of my study. *The Janus Report* shows, however, that 19 percent of very religious men have had sex by age fourteen as compared with 13 percent nonreligious men. But what we don't know is what percentage of these men, now very religious, grew up very religious. Was this rebellion or was it that they had received no sexual instruction? There are too many unknowns here for us to be dogmatic.

Now let us turn to my study of male sexuality to see what it can add to this picture of the relationship between religion and male sexuality.

The Effect of Religion on Raising Boys

The first question I want to address—especially for the benefit of teenage boys' parents—is the effect that religion has on raising boys. The stereotype promulgated by antireligious groups is that overly religious parents mess up their children's sexuality. They teach boys that sex is shameful and that their strong sexual feelings make them the most vile and wicked of all God's creatures.

"My Mom was so uptight she'd leave the dinner table if we boys even joked about sex." This was said by a man on the radio who admits he has

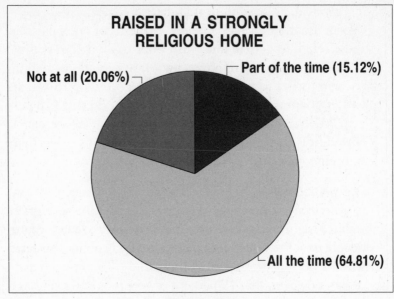

Figure 10.1

serious sexual hang-ups, and blames it all on his overly religious mother. Not once, of course, does he ever say, "But I suppose the time has come for me to take responsibility for my own life and see what I can do to fix it."

Furthermore, I have met as many men who can trace their distorted sexuality to parents who were not religious as those who were. While religious parents may have more restrictions, it is parents who fail to get involved in teaching a healthy sexuality that create many of our problems. It doesn't matter whether negligent parents are religious.

My focus here is, of course, only on how religious factors can form a child's sexual feelings. So to begin let me report on how the men in my sample were raised. Figure 10.1 shows the percentages for those raised "part of the time," "all the time," or "not at all" in a religious home. I took the "not at all" and "all the time" groups and separated them for comparison purposes, discarding the "part of the time" group. My purpose was to see if it makes any difference to a man whether he was raised in a religious home.

How does being raised in a religious home affect your sexuality? Here, of course, I am specifically looking at the Protestant Christian home. I chose to compare those men raised with no religious upbringing to those raised in a religious home all the time on four factors:

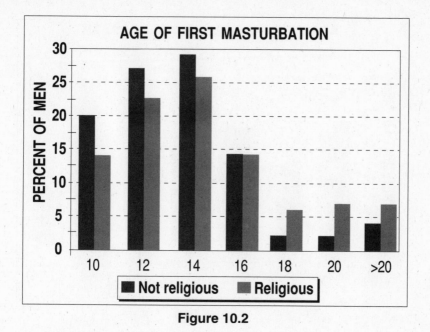

Figure 10.2

1. The effect it had on them when they started masturbating.

2. The effect it had on how early they were exposed to pornography.

3. The effect it had in later life on their sexual attraction to women other than their spouse.

4. The effect it had on current sexual experience.

I could have examined many other effects as well, but these will suffice to show us whether a religious upbringing is all good or all bad.

Age of first masturbation. Figure 10.2 shows a comparison between those men raised with a "not-religious" background versus those raised in a religious home. While the difference is not very great, it is quite consistent for the various age groups. Boys raised in religious homes are *less likely* to start masturbating earlier. For instance, 20 percent of the not-religious background group had started masturbating by age ten, as opposed to 13.5 percent of the religious background group. This difference holds through to age sixteen where the two groups are identical. The religious background

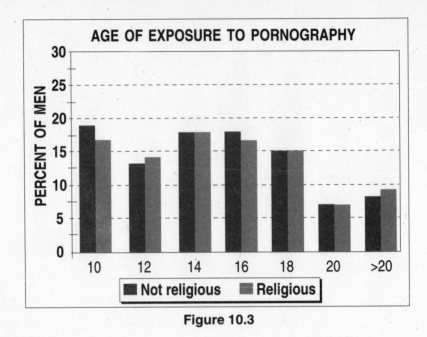

Figure 10.3

boys appear in greater numbers among the boys who start masturbating *after* age sixteen.

Clearly then, a religious home environment raises the age at which boys get into masturbation. Is this a positive effect? Undoubtedly. The earlier a boy starts masturbating, the greater the risk of developing an obsession with it. What is quite clear, however, is that being raised in a religious home doesn't stop boys from masturbating. It just delays it awhile.

What reasons could explain this slowing down? For one thing, boys raised in a religious home are less likely to be exposed to sexually stimulating materials such as magazines or movies. A boy who is surrounded by sex scenes or pictures is likely to develop overt sexual interests earlier and might even experience earlier puberty.

Religious parents might be communicating values that help a boy to restrain his sex drive. They could also be helping their son to find other sublimating outlets, making sexual matters less of a preoccupation. Whatever the reason, the effect though small, is a desirable one.

Age of first exposure to pornography. The results in Figure 10.3 are not as favorable as those regarding first masturbation. Boys raised with a not-religious

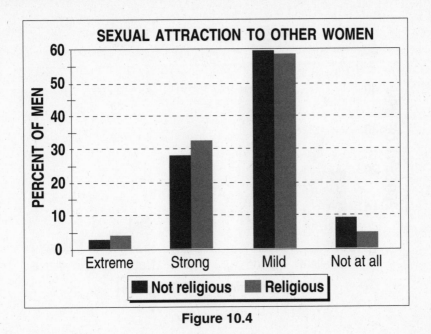

Figure 10.4

background show a slightly greater risk before age ten of first exposure to porn, but thereafter it is remarkably the same as for boys raised in a religious home. In case you're tempted to jump to the conclusion that religious homes have just as much porn in them as nonreligious homes, let me hasten to add that I don't believe this is so.

The effect we are seeing here is the effect of influences *outside* of the home. Before age ten, the home has the major influence; hence nonreligious boys are at greater risk. Thereafter, outside influences take over and boys get pictures from other boys, sneak peeks at late-night movies, and get exposed to porn at other boys' homes.

From age sixteen onward, the age of first exposure is almost identical for the nonreligious and religious background groups. The potential for damage is equal.

Sexual attraction to other women. Does growing up in a strongly religious or Christian home have an effect on how a man is sexually attracted to other women? Figure 10.4 shows a comparison between the not-religious and religious upbringing groups. The categories range from "extremely attracted" to "not attracted at all."

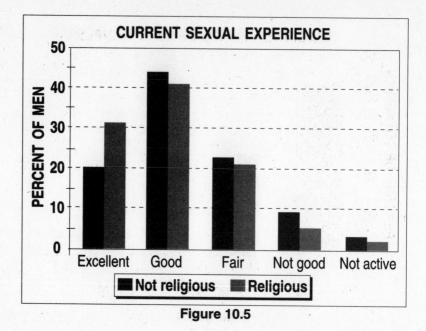

Figure 10.5

At the mild attraction and extreme attraction levels there are no differences between the groups. When we examine those strongly attracted, the religious background group is slightly ahead of the nonreligious group. For the "not at all attracted" category, the religious group is slightly behind.

These differences are not statistically significant, but the religious up-bringing group does show a *slightly* higher tendency to be sexually attracted to other women.

Is this due to the effect of childhood training? Is it because of the more restrictive sexual lives of religious men? I don't know. This is something that needs further study.

Current sexual experience. The final question I want to explore here is whether a religious upbringing has any effect on a man's sexual experience in later life. If it does, is this effect positive or negative? Figure 10.5 shows the comparison.

Clearly, the group of men most likely to describe their current sexual experience as excellent are those who were raised all the time in a strongly Christian home. Around 31 percent said this, whereas only 20 percent of men raised with a nonreligious background described their current experience as excellent.

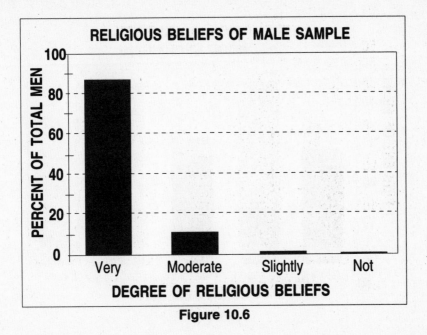

Figure 10.6

Consistent with this, but at the other end, more nonreligious upbringing men are likely to say that their current sexual experience is not good.
In between, the "good" or "fair" groups are about equally represented.

I believe one can say, therefore, that having a strongly Christian upbringing is not detrimental to a man's sexual satisfaction as an adult. If
anything, such a man is more likely to have an excellent experience.

Why is this? It is very possible that the other values communicated in
a deeply Christian home such as love, respect for women, care for the whole
family, and an essentially high standard of morality have positive effects
on a man's adult sexuality. I know that Christian men generally make
better husbands. Perhaps they are more caring, giving lovers as well.
Whatever it is, I'm all for fostering it.

The Effect of Religion on Current Sexual Experience

Religious upbringing is only one factor in the interplay between sex
and religion. Around a third (35 percent) of my sample of men were
raised in either a nonreligious or only partly religious home but are now
fairly religious themselves. How do they, together with those men raised

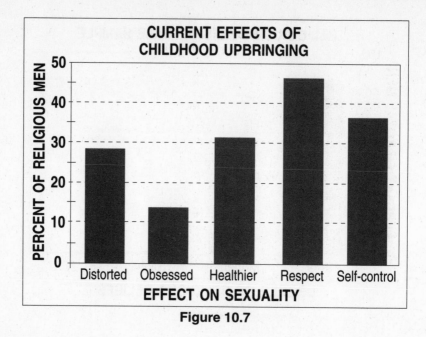

Figure 10.7

in a religious home, view the relationship between their current religious beliefs and their sexuality?

To begin with, Figure 10.6 presents the degree of religious belief in my male sample. Most (86 percent) describe themselves as very religious. Their religious affiliations are predominantly Protestant conservative (85 percent). The rest are either liberal, Catholic, Jewish, or nonreligious. For my analysis here I have examined only those males who currently see themselves as either very religious or moderately religious. This comprises 96 percent my total sample.

How do these men, currently religious, view the effect of their upbringing, whether it was religious or not? What harmful or healthy present-day characteristics do they attribute to their upbringing?

Figure 10.7 is a summary of responses to this question. Around 28 percent reported that their upbringing "distorted" their sexuality. This is tied back to the high preponderance of families in which little, if any, accurate information on sexuality is provided. Around 14 percent of the men blamed their obsessional sexuality on their upbringing.

On the positive side we have higher percentages. Around 31 percent said their childhood helped them to become sexually healthier, 37 percent said it taught them greater self-control, and 46 percent said they

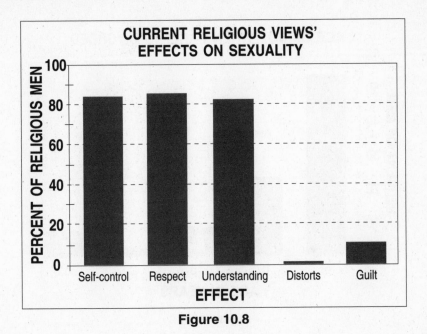

Figure 10.8

learned a greater respect for women than they would otherwise have developed. The positives far outweigh the negatives.

How do the religious views of men influence their current sexuality? See Figure 10.8. Here again, the positives far outweigh the negatives. About 82 percent of the religious men reported that it helps them to achieve greater sexual self-control, 82 percent a greater respect for women, and 81 percent a greater understanding of the role sex plays in human life. These are fairly consistent percentages.

About 18 percent of the religious men (one man in five) blamed their religious views as not being helpful in the area of sexuality. This group of men is probably the least sexually happy of all. Less than 1 percent of the religious men, however, reported that their religious views distorted sexuality and only 6 percent reported that it made them feel a lot of guilt over sex.

Because divorce is so common, even in Christian and deeply religious circles, I wanted to determine whether this played any role in influencing a boy's sexuality. Only 11 percent of my sample reported that their parents did divorce while they were growing up. This is well below the national average, which means that most of the men came from homes free of divorce. This doesn't mean they were happy homes, just that there was no divorce.

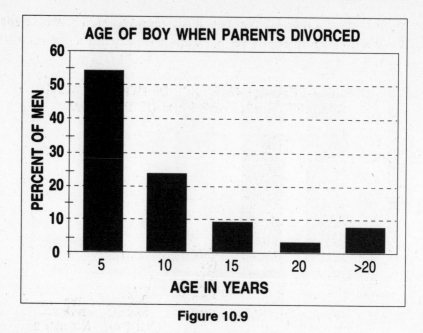

Figure 10.9

The age at which these men experienced their parents' divorce is shown in Figure 10.9. Most of the men whose parents divorced did so when the boys were five or under (54 percent). By age ten it had dropped to 24 percent.

Most of these men experienced their parents' divorce very early in their lives. How has this affected their current sexual experience? Amazingly little. Separating those men whose parents divorced from those whose parents did not divorce and comparing the quality of their current sexual experiences, I came up with Figure 10.10. The two groups follow each other quite closely, seldom differing by more than 2 percent. Experiencing divorce as a child may have other consequences on boys but it doesn't seem to affect the quality of their sexuality later in life.[9]

One last fact concerns the sexual attraction that some men—even deeply religious ones—feel toward other men. While I have deliberately focused this study on heterosexual men, I know from my work as a clinical psychologist that even exclusively heterosexual men are capable of some sexual feelings toward other men. I wanted to know how common this is.

Please note that this is not a report on the incidence of homosexual orientation in general, but only on whether or not heterosexual men have *any* sexual feelings toward other men.

Figure 10.11 presents the results. Most (91 percent) of the religious men in my sample reported never having any sexual feelings or attraction toward other men. Only 4.7 percent of the men reported some "slight" sexual attraction. From the notes accompanying their questionnaires I

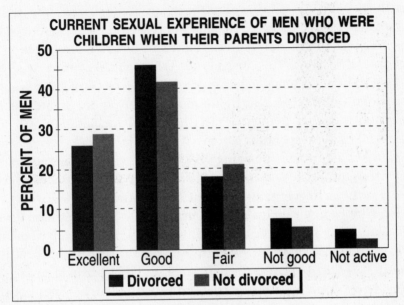

Figure 10.10

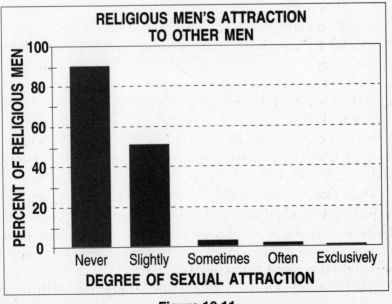

Figure 10.11

gleaned that this meant they had some mild intrigue with other men's penises or bodies, or became slightly aroused at male nudity. Only 3.3 percent reported that they sometimes were sexually attracted to other men. It may have been just a single episode or an attraction to only one person. They insisted they are heterosexual in orientation and often described the "sometimes" as situational. Around 1 percent reported often feeling attracted and 0.27 percent exclusively so. This group, representing a total of 1.27 percent of my religious group of men, could be considered as either homosexual or bisexual; this figure more closely approximates recent studies of homosexual frequencies in the general population.

Several of the respondents in my study spoke of once being homosexual in behavior but now being satisfied and adjusted heterosexuals. One of the untold stories about male sexuality is the number of men who are to some degree sexually attracted to other men but who have achieved happy heterosexual marriages. I have worked in therapy with many such men. They have children, wonderful marital relationships, and exciting sex lives. They wouldn't change it for anything. While they still feel the attraction to their same sex, they are able to use this interest to establish appropriate friendships with men, but they confine their sexual expressions to their wives.

This is no different than what purely heterosexual men have to learn to do with their sexual feelings for other women. Homosexual men who have adjusted to a heterosexual lifestyle still continue to be aware of their feelings for other men. They just make the choices that help them focus their sexual feelings on their female partner. It's a matter of choice.

I emphasize this point here because many men who have same-sex attraction cannot entirely undo this attraction by themselves. Some have achieved remarkable freedom through Christian resources, but others have not. I liken it to learning to ride a bicycle. Once you've learned it, no one can take that ability away from you. Once you have opened up same-sex sexual feelings, seldom can it just be zapped away, even with the deepest of religious experiences.

One can learn to change behavior, however. Just as the heterosexual learns this in order to stay monogamous, so a man with sexual attractions to other men can choose to live a heterosexual lifestyle. Like all the rest of us, he exercises choices to focus his sexuality heterosexually.

Sex, the Christian Male, and the Clergy

Nothing divides modern religious groups, especially Catholics and Protestants, more than sex. No more challenging problem faces Christianity as we move to a new millennium. From the troubled boy who suffers painful guilt because he masturbates, through premarital intercourse, teenage pregnancy, sexual violence toward women, homosexuality, and extramarital affairs, Christianity is under pressure. Some want to slacken restrictions. Others want to embrace a more conventional morality.

Theologically, Protestants have resolved their schizophrenic feelings about sex. Sex is a natural instinct that must be accepted and enjoyed, but sex can also become repressed and produce perversion and harm. So we travel a two-lane highway. One lane carries the traffic of reproduction, the other the quieting of lust.

But the tug of war is still here. Men who want to be good and decent find themselves pushed and pulled by lustful urges and aspirations to transcend these urges. For most Christian men, the control of sex is an ongoing challenge that takes far more energy than it deserves. The toughest problem Christian men have to face is how they feel about their sexuality.[10] And since the Bible doesn't spell out a concise theory of sexuality, many have to work out one for themselves. Unfortunately, they don't always do a good job.

Meanwhile, an epidemic of sexual indiscretions amongst the clergy is hitting the headlines.

The philandering pastor is a familiar figure in American fiction. Many novelists have found success by critically looking at the human side of pastors and priests. Elmer Gantry is just one of many who have led the pack, though real-life makes Elmer look pale. Novels often make fun of religious piety and try to show its hypocrisies. But real-life stories of lechers in clerical clothing eclipse fiction. Victims are shamed, congregations are embarrassed, and only a few clergy are severely dealt with. Protestants and Catholics are reeling from embarrassment.

There are no national statistics on the sexual misconduct by clergy. My research reports anywhere from 12 percent to 30 percent of the clergy have had some inappropriate sexual encounter.

Why all this concern about clergy? Aren't they human like the rest of us? Yes they are. But ordinary folk have a right to expect clergy not to use their positions of influence and power to obtain sexual gratification either with women or children. We trust them with our nearest and dearest. They ought to be honorable and worthy of this trust.

There is nothing new about ministers who think ordination is a license to cheat on their wives or religious orders. Henry Ward Beecher, the great preacher of the nineteenth century, was ruined following an affair. But there is growing concern today about local pastors who seduce or who are seduced by parishioners who rely on them for spiritual guidance in troubled times. Such betrayal strikes at the very heart of pastoral calling. A church is completely ruined by such betrayal by its leader.

Who is at risk? The minister most likely to stray is middle-aged, disillusioned with his calling, neglectful of his own marriage, a lone ranger, isolated from clerical colleagues. Then he meets a woman who needs him.[11]

The pastoral seducer is different from other men because he has the ability to reduce guilt in the follower he seduces. He literally gives her a "guilt-free trip" in the affair. She believes that if he, as pastor, thinks it's okay to have an affair, then it can't be all that sinful. So she succumbs.

Generally speaking, most of the pastors who fall are average, ordinary men. They are not hard-core sex perverts or chronic seducers. They succumb to a special need in a moment of weakness, then live to regret it whether they are found out or not. So let us not be too harsh in our judgment here. These men need remedial therapy, close supervision and accountability, and an opportunity to demonstrate that they can be trusted again.

Some pastors are not taught in their seminaries to recognize the unique feelings encountered in the counseling setting (called *transference* and *countertransference*). They misread these feelings. It makes matters worse if they are lacking in accountability. Finally, in their training, they are not taught to adequately address their sexuality or their unmet sexual needs. They are often blind to their hang-ups and may even be so repressed that they don't see their vulnerable points.

Religious men, more than nonreligious men, don't talk about their sexuality, so they never get an opportunity to be honest with themselves and with God. And if there's no self-honesty, there can be no integration of the sexual side of a man with his spiritual side. He splits, developing two sides to himself that are continually at war.

James wrote: "A double minded man is unstable in all his ways" (James 1:8). He was talking about faith. But I think these words of wisdom also apply to the man who hasn't blended his sexual life with his religious life. This, I believe, is all part of developing a healthy sexuality. And that is the topic for the next and final chapter of this book.

11

Creating a Healthy Sexuality

Listening to a radio program a few months ago, I heard an expert on sexuality say, "Sex is a weakness, not a virtue." He then went on to explain that for the male, sex was like a fire: it will burn whether you like it or not and sometimes where you don't want it to. You can feed it with thoughts and fantasies, or you can starve it by distraction or finding alternative creative and engaging challenges.

Is sex only a weakness? Is there nothing good to be said about it? Is it only and always a problem? Sounds too pessimistic to me. Perhaps it would be more accurate to say that sex only tests and defines our other weaknesses.

You see, I believe sex is a virtue. It is when sex is distorted and corrupted that it is a fault. But it can be something beautiful, virtuous, and good. After all, it is an expression of the deepest form of human love possible. And it is medicine to the body, the emotions, and the soul.

But there is a caveat. Sex, left to define itself, can never become virtuous. A magnificent horse, left in the wild to do its instinctive thing, is unbridled and dangerous. And so is sex, left to itself with no bridling and no boundaries. Every splendid equine quadruped (or horse if you prefer) is the product of careful grooming and training. The same is true of a sexuality that is complete and healthy. Left to itself it becomes rough, rude, and unsafe.

Fostering a Healthy Sexuality for the Future

Otto Rank, the Austrian psychoanalyst famous in the earlier part of this century, described sex as a "disappointing answer to life's riddle."[1] What he means is that too many people try to make sex the biological solution to the ultimate mystery of human existence. For some people, sex becomes all they have to live for, and naturally it becomes a big disappointment. Because of this, I believe that sex education has become a kind of a pretense: we pretend that if we give adequate instruction in the mechanics of sex, we are explaining the mystery and purpose of all there is to sexuality.

Sex education has to get to the secret and enigma of sex or it is not education at all. Otto Rank was right. He said that the sexual conflict we find ourselves in is a universal one. It was there in the past, is with us now, and will be with us in the future. The reason? We don't seem to be able to agree on what the mystery of sex really is!

There is a *natural* guilt that we all feel about recreational sex. Sex for pleasure's sake wants to dominate, and male testosterone wants to rule the day. It wants satisfaction without regard to the consequences. Yet it cannot rule, not in a civilized society. The child and later the adult instinctively knows that if he gives in to his body and its sexual cravings, apart from intentionally wanting to conceive, he will do something wrong. And this deep-seated tension is the source of many sexual problems.

This is the mystery of sex. It is designed for one thing—procreation—but is used primarily for another—pleasure.

When parents just give straightforward biological answers to sexual questions, they do not answer the child's deepest questions at all. He wants to know *why* he has a body, *where* it came from, and *what it means* to be a sexual being.[2] He longs to know about the mystery of it all, of life, reproduction, and ultimately about death. Finally, he needs to know that sex is a delightfully blissful thing and how this fits into the baby-making thing.

One Christian man I know tells me that his single mother went out of her way to tell him about the birds and the bees when he was a child. She used medical terms for female anatomy. In fact, as a boy this man was teased for being "Mr. Doctor." He was a walking medical dictionary.

As he grew older, however, the message he got from his mother was that sex was dangerous. The danger was in intercourse. Don't do it. Everything else was okay, but avoid intercourse like the plague. Reason? "That's where babies come from," she always said with great emotion.

Regrettably her motivation was not to teach abstinence. Her own pain, resulting from a failed teenage marriage (of which he was the product) had distorted the emotions of sex for her. It took this man a long time, well into his adulthood in fact, to get over this bad message.

Modern-day sex education goes one step further down the slippery slope. To solve the problem of teenage pregnancy, it tries to teach birth control, but only the mechanics of birth control. It teaches nothing about the miracle of conception and how little lives are brought into being, even how they were conceived in a moment of bliss. The origin of the problem is seen to be only in the mechanics of premarital sex, and as long as we think of the problem only in terms of its mechanics we will never solve it.

What's wrong with teaching birth control? Nothing. We must teach it. It's what we *don't* teach that is the problem. We don't teach boys and girls what it means to be sexual and the responsibilities that go with it. Instead, we teach sexuality by trying to eradicate any sense of shame associated with premarital sex. The logic used by this modern approach is as follows: Teenage pregnancy is a problem. Birth control is the solution. Shame is the barrier to effective protection. So let us eliminate the shame, take away any embarrassment about obtaining a condom, and we've fulfilled our obligation. We've taught them all they need to know about sexuality.

Are all sexual choices morally neutral? Should there be no shame? No guilt? Where does a young boy learn about healthy guilt? Where does he learn decency and respect for a woman's right to say no?

And by the way, don't assume that all teens are sexually active. I think that much public policy on sex education makes this assumption, and it is not correct. Ask teenagers yourself. They are offended by adults who assume that just because they are boy or girl crazy that all they want is sex. Some may be active, but not all are. So why dump a lot of sexual mechanics on teens who are not and don't want to be sexually active.

What healthy instruction should they get? What about, "How do I make morally right choices?" or, "What should I look for in a mate?" For those of strong religious persuasion another important consideration is, "What does the Bible teach about sex?" The Bible teaches very little about the mechanics of sex but has a lot to say about the mystery of life and childbearing. It is partly because we have neglected those vital issues that we are in trouble.

Guidelines for Healthy Sex Education

I'd like to offer some practical suggestions on teaching the basics of sex. To begin with, by all means give your children all the factual data you can about the physiology and mechanics of sex. Don't wait until puberty before you do so because your son will already have learned it all from other sources by then.

What's wrong with letting him learn about sex on the streets? Because he will probably receive distorted information filtered through myriad screens of fantasy and childish assumption. Sexuality formed by information shared between boys or gleaned from underground pornography is bound to be warped.

Talk about sex early. Whenever the subject naturally arises, talk about it, just as if you were telling your kids about how to brush their teeth or to say please or thank you. The more natural you can make these discussions the healthier will be your instruction.

Don't worry about telling your children too much. They won't process information they're not ready for anyway. Telling more than necessary helps to set the stage for the next level of talking, and it helps parents to be approachable.

Use correct terms. Toddlers should learn to use the correct terms for all body parts. After all, they learn knee and hand. Why is it different for the genitals? Why are we embarrassed to say "penis" instead of "weenie"? By using cute words we really teach our children that these parts are secretive or different.

Give honest answers to questions about sex. If your five-year-old asks about intercourse, using our most popular slang word for it, while the boss and his wife are having dinner at your home, don't jump on him with a "How dare you! Get to your room!" response. Be nonreactive, calm, and mature. Kids do this sort of thing. A healthy response is, "That's a very good question. We'll discuss it later when we have time." Believe me, this will make a better impression on your boss than overreaction.

Don't panic in unexpected situations. If you catch your three-year-old playing doctor, a five-year-old mimicking masturbation, a seven-year-old with an erection, or a ten-year-old pouring over a porn magazine, don't panic. The less fuss you make, the better. These are often developmental phases and don't indicate that you are failing as a parent. Children are naturally inquisitive about sex, and such normal sex play is generally harmless. It's your reaction that can do the harm. *Never shame a child over sex.*

Never punish a child for masturbating. I mean NEVER! Boys will experiment, and girls may too. Criticizing or humiliating a child over masturbation can permanently harm his or her sexuality. "Guide and teach" should be our motto, not "punish and criticize." How would you like your son to learn about masturbation? Your choice is twofold: from other boys or yourself.

I recall a client who, when he was very young, in the third grade I believe, was invited by another boy at his church to go into the bathroom so he could show him "the feeling." The other boy began to masturbate and invited my client to join him. My client was pre-ejaculatory, but he mimicked the other boy, going through all the motions. Sure enough, there was "the feeling," and he liked it! Soon he was doing it regularly. At that time he attached no fantasies to it. Even though he had no semen to ejaculate, it still gave him a tremendous thrill.

But in the months that followed his secret search for the feeling literally wore the skin off his penis. The feeling was so overwhelming that even the pain of bruised skin couldn't stop him from trying to get it. And since he couldn't ejaculate, he never, ever climaxed so that the feeling could reach satisfaction and subside. He just kept on going and going. For him, the habit of excessive masturbation became established very early, and it was something he regretted later in life.

The problem, basically, was that he received no instruction as to what was going on. If someone had told him that masturbating so much before you can ejaculate will only cause harm, he might have waited until he was older. But no one talked to him. He needed some early lessons in self-control.

The self-control we teach should not only emphasize "don't overdo it," but also "watch what and how you fantasize." Control of access to pornography is crucial. Provide healthy, instructional sex materials (even though these will also be stimulating to a boy) rather than allow access to raunchy, women-distorting, male-dominated pornography.

Is There a Healthy Shame?

While we as parents and teachers should never shame a child, every child will need to develop a certain degree of shame surrounding his or her sexuality. If we didn't have some shame, we'd all walk around naked and copulate in public places.

This healthy shame is what sets us apart from animals. We need privacy for some human activities, and sex is at the top of the list. Sex has to be private for us. Healthy shame is designed to protect the functions of sex. It fosters the love of one woman, monogamy, and most important of all, other women's freedom from being harassed. If sex were not private we would not be able to maintain a monogamous society.

Shame protects us. Someone has said that it even protects our genitals because it forces us to cover them. There is no culture, no matter how primitive, that doesn't have some of this shame. Even where the climate is hot all year round and nudity is considered natural, private genitals will be covered most of the time. For good health and protection a covering is needed because these are our most sensitive and vulnerable body parts.

The need for covering is not only the product of our Victorian prudishness, but comes from a source deep within us. There exists in all of us an essential intrinsic sexual morality. Some animals have a bit of this, but for them it's instinctive. They stay committed to one partner for life. Many primitive cultures do the same. The reason is that our fantastic mind knows at a deep level that this is the decent thing to do. The same is true with the privacy of sex.

So it is not just the taboos of our society that force us to form this healthy sense of shame but something incorporated into our whole personality. I believe it is God-given for our good. And it is this healthy sense of shame, coming out of whatever basic sense of decency still resides in all of us, that we need to foster in our children as well.

I say "foster" because its basic ingredients are there. But I really mean we must teach it. Why? Because it is essential to sexual self-control. Without it my wife and daughters would not be safe from the hungry sexual appetites of men all around.

This healthy shame is not only a "must-not" kind of shame but also an "ought-to" kind. That I must not view women only as sex objects is right. But I ought to seek the welfare of all women even if they are not sexually attractive to me. This is equally important.

This healthy sense of shame develops when we teach children, especially our boys:

- To respect girls (and women) for being persons and not sex objects
- That girls have a right to say no
- That sex is a private behavior
- That sexual language, especially swearing, can be abusive to women
- That a person who chooses to abstain from inappropriate sexual activity is quite normal and may even have more character than one who doesn't
- That an unbridled sexual urge is always dangerous and abnormal
- That to take someone else you know and use her in your sexual fantasies is a violation of her rights

We must go further in sexually educating our boys than just teaching them the biological elements of sex. We need to form a healthy sense of privacy, respect, and the tender elements of this, the most intimate of human interactions.

What Is a Healthy Male Sexuality?

How can one tell if one's sexuality is healthy? This is not as easy to answer as one would imagine. We could ask questions like:

- How much do you depend on fantasy for sexual arousal?

- Do you have to masturbate in addition to sex to satisfy your needs?

- How do you view an attractive woman? Do you mentally undress her?

- What sexual thoughts do you tend to fill your mind with?

- How often do you think about sex?

These would all be legitimate questions, directly relevant to sexual healthiness. But is there a central issue or a core test of healthiness? I think there is. I came across it years ago in a book by Oswald Schwarz, an Austrian physician who later worked in England and became an expert in human sexuality. He states that *the acid test of a healthy sexuality is "the ability to produce an effective sexual response at the appropriate time and when the right conditions are fulfilled."*[3]

There are three aspects to this core test of how a man's healthy sexuality is. It must be: (1) an effective sexual response, (2) at the appropriate time and toward the right person, and (3) when the right conditions are fulfilled.

An effective sexual response. Having no sexual response, unless there is a biological reason for this, is not a healthy response. Healthiness includes having an *effective* sexual reflex.

In therapeutic circles these days there is a lot of concern being expressed about what is becoming known as the "yuppie disease." What is it? It's impotence at thirty. Young, healthy, and successful otherwise-virile men just cannot perform sexually.

The underlying problem is stress. To be able to work, our bodies draw heavily on the sympathetic system, which gives us energy and keeps us up and running. For sex, one resorts to the parasympathetic system. It calms us down and sends the signals needed for arousal and erection. Since the two systems can't work at the same time, one has to stop so the other can take over. Stress is the real enemy of sexual satisfaction, and any male whose sympathetic system won't switch off will suffer from impotence.

The solution? Relaxation. Lots of it. Don't work so hard, and stay away from alcohol. Drowning your worries with alcohol will only drown your libido as well.

There are other factors that can sabotage a man's sexual response. One of them is just a plain, old-fashioned, hang-up with sex. Sometimes sexual hang-ups have to do with a man's view of his dimensions or the fact that he has premature ejaculations. Men need sexuality to make them whole persons. This is not the same as saying that men need sex. This is another matter. In fact, when men only need sex and sex only without the accompaniments of love, tenderness, and relationship, they have a disfigured sexuality. When men need sex only for pleasure and relief of physical tension, you have a neuroticized sexuality.

At the appropriate time and toward the right person. This means that a man is able to focus his sexual arousal on his chosen partner. This way he limits his arousal toward other women. For a man to be healthy he *must* be able to restrict his arousal to appropriate people—or preferably to one person, his partner.

Let me take an extreme case to illustrate this. Men who respond with sexual arousal to children *do not have a healthy sexuality*. No respectable group in our culture sees such an attraction as healthy. I know that some men feel this attraction, for whatever reason, but don't act on it. Those who do need to seek treatment right away because they are dangerous.

Sexual arousal "at the appropriate time and toward the right person," then, not only means that one does not feel sexually attracted to children, including one's own children (even if they are grown-up), but it also means that one is able to limit and control one's sexual attraction toward other men's wives. This means that men should be able to control arousal in the workplace and socially.

Men who fail the test of healthy sexuality because they become aroused at an inappropriate time or toward the wrong person need to face up to the fact that their sexual drive may be out of control. Such a response is common and is certainly the underlying problem that defines most of the sexual perversions.

When the right conditions are fulfilled. More marital unhappiness is caused by this third and final test of sexual healthiness than anything else I know. This touches on a basic problem with male sexuality. It doesn't always wait for the right conditions; it is not always patient enough to ensure that the right conditions are fulfilled.

Males hormones make climax the whole aim and ambition of the sex drive. But in order to satisfy deeper psychological needs, a man needs to learn how to be romantic, tender, and nurturing. Without these, sex is a hollow event. Women universally complain that men want only one thing, and it is always the same thing. To satisfy a female's sexual responsiveness, a man often has to postpone his climax. That goes against his sexual nature *unless* he has learned not to be so impulsive.

For the healthy male, then, this natural urgency has to be brought under control, and we have the means to do this through our wonderful brains, which ultimately control the sexual response. The brain is the executive organ for all humans, even of the highly aroused male. And when it knows what is right, it can do right. This means that the right conditions can be learned.

Working against this control is the male's tendency to split off sex from love, thus losing the potential for finding a deep level of satisfaction from sex. When a man sees sex as being devoid of the love connection, reducing it to mere biological release, that man robs himself of true ecstasy.

Oswald Schwarz illustrates this splitting in the male with a story about a very distinguished elderly gentleman who "honored" his parlor maid by inviting her into his bed.[4] Afterward the young lady tried to kiss him good-bye. The gentleman reacted indignantly, saying that what she was trying to do was "disgusting."

Taken aback, the maid left as fast as she could. Her need for intimacy and his need for sex did not meet. I have talked to scores of wives who have tried to get a kiss from a just-satisfied husband and have just as quickly been pushed away. A kiss is disgustingly intimate to many males once the sexual drive is satisfied.

So male sexuality has to learn both how to create the right conditions for its fulfillment and to confine itself if the conditions are not right. The right conditions also include certain moral limits. Having sex with a prostitute is not a right condition for sex, and men who prefer this cannot be said to have a healthy sexuality. The same can be said of extramarital or even premarital relations.

Immorality in sex never pays off; it can never define a healthy sexuality. Immoral sexual behavior has a deleterious effect on a man's sexuality, but more than this, immorality deprives women of their natural value and dignity. An immoral act almost always implies that a woman's rights are being violated. A husband who has an affair with another woman is violating his wife's rights.

The problem is who defines this morality? Where does one go to find out what is right and what is wrong, what is healthy and what is destructive? I have refrained throughout this book from pushing a specifically Christian or biblical morality at my reader, not because I don't believe in it but because I hoped to be able to show that there are very practical reasons why we need a high standard of morality to help us define sexuality.

Ultimately it is our morals that define what is and what is not healthy. Morality determines *when* the conditions for sexual arousal are right. And I happen to believe that the conventional morality of the Christian faith is neither arbitrary nor capricious. When we ignore it, it is our peril.

Strategies for Sexual Control

There is absolutely no doubt in my mind that we have to resort to higher resources to help us regulate our sexual urges. I would call these "psycho-spiritual" factors. I know that just using the word *spiritual* could turn some readers off, but hear me out before you tune me out. A combination of psychological strategies and spiritual dependence and resources are *the only effective tools we have for governing the sexual urge*. Every form of recovery ever devised uses this combination of psychological and spiritual resources. I wish it were easier, but it isn't. There's no pill that can take away the sexual drive. Raging hormones burn away any feeble barriers or demolish any unorganized attack on them. In light of this, I suggest two sets of strategies, one psychological and one spiritual, for dealing with sexual control.

Psychological strategies. Three psychological strategies are available.

1. *Conscious control and distractions.* The first level at which we can exercise control is at the conscious level. We can reason with ourselves. We have choices. I can choose whether or not to buy a pornographic magazine, indulge a sexual fantasy, or turn away from a temptation. We do this by using our reasoning ability.

Sometimes this approach is called *self-talk*. We converse with ourselves and try to reason some sense into our behavior. Reasoning with ourselves is always an option, no matter how out of control we feel.

Reason has to be accompanied by *distraction*. For distraction to work you need to have a competing activity already planned that will capture your attention and distract you from your sexual preoccupations. Hobbies, sports, friends, or even memories of pleasant events can do it.

Take Roy, for instance. He's obsessing about a hidden pornographic magazine. He sneaked it home in his briefcase, hoping his wife wouldn't notice. Now he feels a strong flow of sex hormones as he recalls the few glimpses he had of it before he hurriedly hid it beneath some papers. Roy wishes his wife would hurry up, finish cleaning the kitchen, and leave for her evening ladies meeting so he can have some privacy to indulge his lusting appetite. He's restless. His wife notices and remarks on it. He gets mad and storms off to watch television. The sexual excitement actually increases for Roy when he gets mad at his wife. It swamps his feelings of guilt.

Then Roy remembers that he had promised himself he would try to break his dependence on pornography and remembers the distraction technique he had been taught at a men's meeting at church. He goes to the bedroom to catch his wife before she leaves.

"I think I'll go down to the gym and work out for a bit," he says. "Haven't been there in several days." An hour later Roy has worked up quite a sweat. The workout has helped distract his sexual urge for porn and has refocused him on more important issues.

Without a distraction Roy would have found it almost impossible to escape the attraction of the pornography he had acquired. The next day he trashes the magazine.

2. *Uncovering unconscious forces*. For many men, the driving force behind their ungovernable sexuality originates deeper than their hormones. It arises from somewhere in their unconscious. Childhood abuse, premature exposure to sex or sexually stimulating material, or a host of unmet psychological needs can all be exerting a pressure for some inappropriate sexual experience. And these men are without any awareness of these unconscious forces.

We probably all have some unconsciously repressed sexual material that breaks through to shape our present sexual preferences. The more we understand and can recognize these unconscious forces, the healthier we are. Often just bringing them into conscious awareness is enough to free us from their power to influence us.

There is little by way of self-help that I can point to here. Psychotherapy is almost always essential. It takes some expert probing to get at deeply repressed material, though be careful to whom you entrust the probing of your unconscious.

There is a growing awareness that some therapists have a penchant for uncovering harmful memories of events that never actually occurred. We call this the "false memory syndrome." Many innocent parents, uncles, friends, and teachers have been blamed by overzealous therapists who see sexual abuse behind every neurosis or sexual dysfunction. As one who trains clinical psychologists I am appalled at the absurd arrogance of some incompetent psychologists and counselors who overinterpret the slightest bit of evidence that hints at abuse; so beware!

3. *Sublimation.* We discussed sublimation earlier, and people have known about it for a long time. Freud helped us to see its value in coping with unacceptable impulses. It is here that an instinctive drive like sex, when out of control or lacking in fulfillment, can be transformed into a higher, equally satisfying but nonsexual activity. Sexual instincts are often sublimated by satisfying work or by serving other people in a sacrificial way. Just how the brain accomplishes this is not quite clear, but it does.

By and large, sublimation is viewed to be healthy, but it has its risks.

For instance, a young man who is sexually attracted to boys may find that being a priest involved in youth work is fulfilling enough to sublimate his attraction. But being exposed to the very source of his unhealthy attraction may, in fact, feed his problem, working against the sublimation. So it is better for this young man to seek his sublimation elsewhere. Being a priest to the elderly may not be as effective as youth ministry in helping sublimation, but it may be the only safe alternative.

Many men have been drawn to work that they feel will help them control their sexual urges only to find that it has increased their vulnerability. This is one of the reasons why I strongly advocate that men going into the ministry need to confront and heal their sexuality while they are still in seminary. A pastor who tries to sublimate a strong sex drive through Christian service may find that the work only makes him or her more vulnerable.

Unless you can find sublimating relief in areas unrelated to your sexual problem, forget about this approach. You are only fooling yourself if you think you can achieve control of your fire while pouring oil on it.

Spiritual strategies. Three spiritual strategies are available.

1. *Acknowledge your lack of power to control your sexual urges.* This strategy is the cornerstone of all recovery groups. Any approach that uses

the twelve-step method requires it. Why? Because, quite frankly, the average American male is powerless against the mighty forces of testosterone. The human mind, as marvelous as it is, has its limitations. Some can try all the will power they can muster, all the reasoning strategies they can devise, and all the distractions imaginable, and they will still lose the battle.

Sexual desire is one of the strongest drives in the human body. And there comes a time when you have to say, "I can't control it anymore—it's beyond me. So God, give me the strength I need to cope with my sexual urges." This is not the prayer of a weakling but the cry of an honest, determined man who wants to be decent.

Now let's get a very important point straight about *how* God helps us when we pray this prayer. It is not that God takes over our bodily functions or that He throws a few switches and passes control of our brain's functions to some heavenly console. If He did that we would be mere robots—automatons. There could never be a "well done thou good and faithful servant" at the end because we wouldn't have done anything at all. It would have been done for us.

I stress this point because so many Christian people seem to think that surrendering a problem to God means they don't have to do any more work. It's like when you were a little child and something you prized broke and you started crying. What did your father do? He said, "Here, give it to me and I will fix it for you." We gladly surrendered it, then sat back and waited for the return of our restored prized object.

Does God work this way? Sometimes. Yes, I've known cases where the sufferer has not had an ounce of strength or any ability to help himself, and God has gently said, "Here, give your problem to Me and I will fix it for you." But is this always how God works? Absolutely not.

Yes, God *does* answer our prayer for empowerment, but more often than not He points us back toward what we have to do or toward some resource we didn't think we had. He helps us muster a little more courage to take a stand or resist temptation. Occasionally, He might just work a special miracle and you will feel a release from your sexual prison. It is always miraculous to suddenly discover He is beside you, keeping you company as you work through some pain, grasp some insight, or turn your back on a temptation.

When you acknowledge that you have reached the end of your resources and reach out for God's help, don't be surprised if He doesn't zap your problem and take it instantly away. But don't expect God to relieve you of your responsibility to change. He doesn't work that way. But what He does is so much more meaningful. He shows us where and how to grow, points us to resources within and without ourselves, and then gives us what we need to act on these resources.

2. *Appeal to resources outside yourself.* One of the ways God makes a difference in our lives is that He inspires people to help other people. This is what Galatians 6:2 tells us: "Bear ye one another's burdens, and so fulfill the law of Christ." Nowhere is the need to bear each other's burdens greater than in the area of human sexuality. God has given us each other as helpers and guides so that we might teach each other how to be healthier.

The same idea of mutual help is set forth at the beginning of 2 Corinthians where Paul tells us that God, who is the God of all comfort, "comforts us in all our troubles, so that we can comfort those in any trouble with the comfort we ourselves have received from God" (2 Cor. 1:4 NIV).

I have seldom seen a man with a serious sexual problem fix it by himself. There's just too much that can sabotage one's own healing. We need help from others, and not necessarily professional help, unless the problem is a serious one. Why must we open up to others? There are two important reasons: to keep us honest and to hold us accountable.

I once counseled with a minister who had a serious problem with sexuality for most of his professional life. Behind him were a long string of inappropriate sexual actions that harmed many people. Finally, his life of sex had caught up with him and he was in serious trouble. I asked him, "Why did you not get help for your problem sooner?"

He replied, "I didn't want to tell anyone I had a problem because I knew they would then keep an eye on me."

This is precisely why we should share our problems with others, so they can help us monitor ourselves.

I see the reaching out to a resource outside of yourself as a spiritual action because God's grace can come to you through the help of a friend or an understanding spouse. It can also come through a trained and knowledgeable professional. They are all gifts of God's grace.

"But isn't it enough to just tell God about my problem?" No, it isn't. God knows you better than this. You need to hold yourself accountable to a person as well so you can't play spiritual games! You need to profess a good profession "before many witnesses" (1 Tim. 6:12).

3. *The integration of your whole self into a more balanced life*. All our sexuality needs to be intimately linked with our whole personality. Who we are as sexual beings defines who we are as persons. Too often, however, sex and the self are kept apart—miles apart.

Many men and women have compartmentalized their sexuality in order to maintain any sense of self-respect and dignity. Spiritual men keep their sex in another room so as to limit their guilt and avoid feeling like hypocrites. When they are sexual, they fear they might do and think things they wouldn't consider when not aroused sexually. So they keep sex separated, almost as if it is in another world. This explains why otherwise moral and upright men can have pretty sordid affairs. They have so effectively split off their sexuality that it never dawns on them that they have fractured their personalities. They lack self-integration.

Is this healthy? No, it isn't. Compartmentalized sexuality is dangerous and not conducive to a balanced life. Certainly, you can never feel like a whole person when such splitting is a significant part of your personality. The goal, then, of all sexual wholeness must be the integration of our sexuality into our total personality. It must not be allowed to remain split off.

Moving into Wholeness

The integration of our sexuality into our whole personality is painful, hard work. We have to force ourselves to be ruthlessly honest about who we are in the deep, secret corners of our sexual minds. This process involves being open with a significant other, a willingness to limit the expression of some of our desires, the healing of obvious distortions, and a frank acceptance of our basic sexual makeup. Frankly, without God's guidance and support and the special work of His Spirit, I doubt if we can ever successfully complete this journey toward sexual wholeness.

A friend of mine, Dr. Lewis Smedes, asserts that the gospel affirms that we must strive to achieve this wholeness and integration of our total selves, including our sexuality, into a balanced life. He writes, "But sexuality is not affirmed as an animal dynamic that surges solo in its own arena of hormones and genitalia. . . . The gospel sets the vital springs of biological sexuality into the rapids of personal life. Sexual life is reintegrated into the personal life by the power of the Spirit."[5]

Until we men achieve this integration, our sexuality will always be like a coat of many colors worn on the outside. Pretty, yes. Pleasurable, yes. But deeply satisfying? Never. It is too superficial. It seeks immediate gratification. It lies on the surface of our personalities, adorning our personas but never becoming an integral part of our being. When allowed to remain so, it will always be something we use rather than live.

Who struggles the most to achieve integration? Spiritually sensitive men, of course. Those who desire to live a fault-free life, deeply committed to God. These men struggle the most because they care. Others are content to wear their sexuality as a temporary coat, putting it on or taking it off as their whims dictate. But men who are good and desire to be whole and unblemished can't live this way. They can't stand the hypocrisy of it all.

Without a healthy integration of our sexuality into our total being, it's not possible to be faithful. There will always be the temptation to seek a little more pleasure or one more thrill. If your sexuality is not integral with your morals you will always be tempted to take off your sexual coat too easily and make a bed out of it.

Modern Americans, especially men, evaluate their sexual fulfillment by how good it makes them feel. Sooner or later they discover that their search for the ultimate ecstasy or sexual experience is a hopeless one. Like the pot of gold at the end of the rainbow, it doesn't exist. Extreme sexual gratification is a bottomless pit that can never be totally satisfied. One must be content with the rainbow, which after all, is the real gold.

Sex is not all of life, only a part of it. We need to be saved from making it the be-all and end-all of our existence. We need to be saved to a higher quality of life. To do this we must be prepared to sacrifice our immediate petty gratifications so that the real pleasures of total intercourse involving all of our being can be experienced. God made us sexual. Our sexuality is a joy and a privilege. May we as men find the healthiest pathway to fulfilling this joy.

HINTS FOR CONTROLLING LUST

1. Own up to your lust and admit it is a problem that needs to be controlled. Don't excuse it. Don't rationalize it away. Just be honest with yourself.

2. Don't feed your lust. Cut out anything in your life that feeds it. Don't dwell on thoughts that foster it. Dispose of all sources of stimulation that provoke your lustfulness.

3. Develop alternative diversionary strategies. Find a hobby or activity that you can turn to whenever your feelings of lust become overwhelming.

4. Change your beliefs about sexual lust. Remind yourself that pictures are only pictures, not people, and that you don't have a right to take anyone you desire to bed with you in your imagination.

5. Observe how others who have allowed their lust to go too far have fallen and learn your lesson from their failures, not your own. Prevention is better than cure.

6. Try to find the underlying reason for your lust, beyond just blaming it on your strong sex drive. Lots of men have a strong drive, but are not dominated by lust. Were you love-deprived as a child? Sexually abused? Getting these repressed reasons out into the light can help free you from their hidden power.

7. If you cannot bring lust under control by yourself, get professional help.

Postscript

This, then, is the story of the sexual man. Not a pretty story in some respects. We are facing some serious trends that need to be corrected. Male sexuality needs a lot of repairing before it can claim any semblance of healthiness. It needs to be saved from the direction it is going—a direction that only spells disaster for both men and women.

But it is also not a hopeless story. I was deeply impressed by the many responses I received from Christian men to my questionnaire. They repeatedly encouraged me to tell the whole story from my vantage point. These men represent about as honest and good a group of men as you will find anywhere, but they nearly all said that the male's sex drive is in need of restoration. They helped me to see how their religious practices both hindered and helped them to become healthier and more sexually integrated.

Overall, what I found out about the impact of Christian faith on the formation of a healthy sexuality was more positive than negative. I wouldn't say that I was surprised, but from all my therapeutic work with men like this I did expect them to blame their religious backgrounds more than they did. Most reported that they were healthier in their sexuality because of their faith, not more distorted. Whatever I found to be negative came more from the faulty application of the Christian faith than from the doctrines of faith. It resulted from how the faith was *taught* and *preached*. Not every preacher teaches a healthy faith.

There is no doubt at all in my mind that what the Christian faith teaches is fundamentally healthy and that our human sexuality can be redeemed by it as much as our souls.

We have been set free to experience the joy of our sexuality. We have also been given the resources we need to help us undo the distortions of our sexuality that inevitably will follow from our brokenness and imperfections as humans. This healing is built into God's plan for all humanity. All it takes from us is some cooperation with this plan.

Appendix 1

The Heterosexual Male Experience

(The Survey Used in This Study)

Many men fear that their experience of sexuality may be offbeat or a little different from most other men. The purpose of this study is to find out what men really think about their sexuality and sexual feelings. I want to learn as much as possible about what the average male experience actually is, not what someone would like it to be. On a photocopy of the following survey please answer the questions as honestly as possible. Your frank answers will help all of us understand masculinity at a time when men are becoming increasingly bewildered by the many myths and unrealistic stereotypes of sexuality. We need accurate and reliable information on this important topic, and your contribution will help to clarify a lot of misunderstanding. If you are mailing the questionnaire back to me do not give a return address on the envelope so that your identity will not be known. Thank you for your help.

Dr. Archibald D. Hart

I. BACKGROUND INFORMATION

Age? _____

Marital status? (circle one)
Single / Married / Divorced / Divorced and remarried

Education? (circle highest)
Junior high / High school / College graduate /
Professional degree

Occupation? (Job title or description): _____
_____

II. EARLY SEXUAL EXPERIENCE

1. I believe I reached puberty at _____ years.

2. The earliest age I recall having sexual feelings was _____ years.

3. I first masturbated at age _____ years (zero if never masturbated).

4. By age sixteen, I estimate that I masturbated about _____ times per month (zero if never).

5. My first exposure to X-rated pornographic magazines or movies was at age _____ years (zero if never).

6. I believe that the effect of this early exposure to X-rated material has, in the long run, been (circle one):
Beneficial / Neutral / Destructive / Not exposed

7. I was raised in a strongly religious home (circle one):
Part of my youth / All of my youth / Not at all

8. My instruction in sexuality while growing up was (circle all that apply):
Healthy / Unhealthy   Adequate / Inadequate
Helpful / Unhelpful   Accurate / Distorted

III. PRESENT SEXUAL EXPERIENCE

9. I have been married for _____ years (zero if not currently married).

10. If single, I currently have a sexual partner (circle one):
    Always / Often / Sometimes / Rarely / Never

11. I would rate my current sexual experience as (circle one):
    Excellent / Good / Fair / Not good / Not active

12. I find that my sexual attraction to women other than my partner is (circle one):
    Extremely strong / Strong / Mild / Not at all / Other _____

13. I find it sexually stimulating to fantasize about having sex with someone other than my partner.   Yes / No

14. I estimate that I currently masturbate about _____ times per month (zero if you don't).

15. I masturbate (circle all that apply):
    By myself / With partner / With phone-sex (900 number) /
    With pornography / Other _____

16. My tendency to masturbate makes me feel (circle all that apply):
    Guilty / Shameful / Abnormal / Normal

17. I am able to discuss my masturbation experience with (circle all that apply):
    Pastor, priest, or rabbi / Counselor / Friend / Partner / No one /
    Other _____

18. I believe the reason(s) I masturbate is/are that I (circle one or more):
    Have a strong sex drive / Have an addiction to it / Just a habit /
    No other sexual outlet / Merely enjoy it / Don't masturbate /
    Sex is not available / Feel sexually aroused / Don't know /
    Other _____

19. I fantasize about someone other than my partner during mastur-
    bation or sex (circle one):
    Often / Sometimes / Never / Doesn't apply

20. Most of my sexual fantasies are about (circle one):
    Partner / Friend / Stranger / Fantasy person / Don't know

21. I feel that my sexual needs are being met (circle one):
    Always / Often / Sometimes / Rarely / Never

22. What mostly prevents me from having my sexual needs met is
    (circle one):
    My partner is not ready / Partner is unavailable /
    I am not ready / I am not interested / I don't have a partner /
    Other _____

23. My thoughts turn to sex about once every (circle one):
    Year / Month / Week / Day / Hour / Minute / Never

24. The main source of my sexual arousal is (circle one):
    Partner / Movies / Magazines / Other women / Just happens /
    Don't know / Other _____

25. I have sexual dreams (circle one):
    Rarely / Yearly / Monthly / Weekly / Nightly

26. I have an orgasm in my dreams or sleep (circle one):
    Rarely / Yearly / Monthly / Weekly / Nightly

27. I believe it is physically possible to have sex with someone I
    don't love.   Yes / No

28. I experience a strong sexual desire for someone other than my
    partner (circle one):
    Very often / Often / Sometimes / Rarely / Never.

29. At present my sex drive is (circle one):
    Very strong / Strong / Moderate / Low / Feel no sex drive

30. I feel that pornography is (circle all that apply):
Educational / Helpful / Neutral / Harmful /
Degrading to women / Promotes violence toward women /
Degrades sex / Creates sexual addictions / Distorts sexuality /
Destructive to youth / Other _____

31. I am sexually attracted to other men (circle one):
Never / Slightly / Sometimes / Often / Exclusively

32. I am able to discuss my personal sexual feelings or activities with (circle all that apply):
Parent / Partner / One friend / Several friends / No one

IV. SEXUALITY IN THE WORKPLACE

33. Do you work in a setting where you are in contact with women?
Yes / No

If you don't work with or have contact with women skip to question 41.

34. At work, one or more women are (circle all that apply):
Under my supervision / Of equal rank / My supervisor(s) /
My customers / My vendors

35. Does working around women cause you any sexual arousal? (circle one)
A little / A lot / Not at all

36. If you do experience any degree of arousal around women, how do you feel? (circle one)
It bothers me greatly / Only slightly / Not at all

37. How often do women in your workplace dress provocatively (short skirts, low-cut blouses, tight clothes)?
Never / Sometimes / Often / Always

38. If you are exposed to provocative dress, how do you experience it? (circle all that apply)
    Sexually arousing to me / Enjoyable, but not a problem / Appropriate / Not appropriate / Distracts from my work / Doesn't bother me at all

39. Do you ever encounter any of the following at work? (circle all that apply)
    Overt sexual advances / Subtle sexual advances / Flirtations / Overfriendliness / None of these

40. In your workplace have you ever seen men take inappropriate sexual advantage of women by, for instance, denying them promotion or by other abuse of power?   Yes / No

41. What do you believe about the present laws governing sexual harassment? (circle one)
    Fair to both sexes / Fair only to women / Fair only to men / Not fair at all / Don't know these laws

V. RELIGIOUS BACKGROUND

42. How would you describe your religious beliefs? (circle one or more)
    Very religious / Moderately religious / Slightly religious / Not religious at all

43. What is your religion? (circle one)
    Jewish (liberal) / Jewish (conservative) / Catholic (liberal) / Catholic (conservative) / Protestant (liberal) / Protestant (evangelical) / Protestant (fundamentalist) / New age / Muslim / Buddhist / Other _____

44. Did your parents divorce while you were growing up and what was your age?   No / Yes / At age _____

45. How do you believe your upbringing affects your sexuality?
    (circle all that apply)
    Distorted it / Created unnecessary fears /
    Harmed my relationships with women /
    Caused me to become obsessed with sex /
    Helped me become a healthier person /
    Taught me respect for women / Taught me self-control /
    Other _____

46. How do your current religious views help your sexuality now?
    (circle all that apply)
    Teach me self-control / Teach me respect for women /
    Help me understand the role of sex /
    Feed my sexual desires / Distort sexuality /
    Cause me lots of guilt feelings / Other _____

Please return your completed questionnaire to:
**Dr. Archibald D. Hart
180 N. Oakland Avenue
Pasadena, California 91101**

Appendix 2

Where to Get Help for Sexual Problems

Sex Addicts Anonymous
National Service Organization for S.A.A. Inc.
P. O. Box 70949
Houston, Texas 77270
713-869-4902

Sexaholics Anonymous
Simi Valley, California
805-581-3343

Sexual Compulsives Anonymous
Los Angeles, California, 213-859-5585
New York, New York, 212-439-1123

Sex and Love Addicts Anonymous
Boston, Massachusetts
617-332-1845

Sex Offenders Anomymous – SOANON
Van Nuys, California 91409
818-244-6331

The above programs have groups around the country and should be able to give you a number to call in your locality.

Christian Association for Psychological Studies (CAPS)
Robert R. King, Jr., Ph.D., Executive Secretary
P. O. Box 890279
Temecula, California 92589-0279
909-695-2277
This is a referral service of counselors.

Fuller Psychological and Family Services
The Psychological Center
180 North Oakland Avenue
Pasadena, California 91101
818-584-5555
Counselors are available by appointment.

Biola Counseling Center
13800 Biola Avenue
La Mirada, California 90639
310-903-4800
Counselors are available by appointment.

Notes

Chapter 1   Male Sexuality—The Untold Story

1. Alfred C. Kinsey, W. Pomeroy, and C. Martin, *Sexual Behavior in the Human Male* (Philadelphia: Saunders, 1948).

2. Kinsey, Pomeroy, and Martin, *Sexual Behavior in the Human Female* (Philadephia: Saunders, 1953).

3. Clifford Linedecker, *Children in Chains* (New York: Everest House, 1981).

4. W. H. Masters and V. E. Johnson, *Human Sexual Response* (Boston: Little, Brown, 1966).

5. Barry McCarthy, *What You Still Don't Know about Male Sexuality* (New York: Crowell, 1977).

6. Bernie Zilbergeld, *Male Sexuality: A Guide to Sexual Fulfillment* (Boston: Little, Brown, 1978).

7. Herb Goldberg, *The New Male: From Self-destruction to Self-care* (New York: William Morrow, 1979).

8. Samuel S. Janus and Cynthia L. Janus, *The Janus Report on Sexual Behavior* (New York: Wiley and Sons, 1993).

Chapter 2   Am I Normal?

1. "Sexual Desire," *U.S. News and World Report*, 6 July 1992, 62.

2. Ibid.

3. Oswald Schwarz, *The Psychology of Sex* (London: Penguin, 1958), 16.

4. "Sexual Desire," 64.

5. Ibid., 62.

Chapter 3   Why Male Sexuality Goes Wrong

1. James D. Weinrich, *Sexual Landscapes* (New York: Charles Scribner's Sons, 1987), 9.

2. Bernie Zilbergeld, *Male Sexuality* (Boston: Little, Brown 1978), 2.

3. Ibid., 4.

4. S. Y. Imopekai, "Attainment of Puberty and Secondary Sexual Characteristics in Some Rural and Urban Nigerian Adolescents," *Nigerian Journal of Guidance and Counseling*, August 1986, 48–55.

5. Anonymous, "An Anatomy of Lust," *Leadership*, Fall 1982, 31.

Chapter 4   How Men Think about Sex

1. Herb Goldberg, *The New Male* (New York: Signet Books, 1979), 101.

2. Susan Crain Bakos, *What Men Really Want* (New York: St. Martin's Press, 1990), 75.

Chapter 5   What Men Really Want from Sex

1. Sandra Crichton, "Sexual Correctness. Has it Gone Too Far?" *Newsweek*, 25 October 1993, 52–56.

2. Ibid., 54.

3. Bernie Zilbergeld, *Male Sexuality* (Boston: Little, Brown, 1978), 360.

4. Ibid., 362.

5. Richard Von Kroft-Ebing, *Psychopathic Sexualis* (London: Mayflower-Dell, 1965), 17.

Chapter 6   Why Men Love/Hate Pornography

1. Beatrice Faust, *Women, Sex and Pornography* (New York: McMillan, 1980), 3.

2. Neil M. Malamuth and Edward Donnerstein, *Pornography and Sexual Agression* (New York: Academic Press, 1984), 7.

3. Ibid., 7.

4. John Bales, *APA Monitor*, November 1993, 7.

5. Malamuth and Donnerstein, *Pornography and Sexual Agression*, 8.

6. Samuel S. Janus and Cynthia L. Janus, *The Janus Report on Sexual Behavior* (New York: Wiley and Sons, 1993), 31.

Chapter 7   Teenage Sexuality

1. Thomas Edwards Brown, *A Guide for Sex Education of Youth* (New York: Association Press, 1968), 34.

2. Janus and Janus, *The Janus Report*, 21.

3. Ibid., 22.

4. Ibid.

5. W. H. Masters, V. E. Johnson, and Robert C. Kolodny, *Human Sexuality* (Glenview, Ill.: Scott, Foresman, 1988), 237.

6. June M. Reinish, *The Kinsey Institute New Report on Sex* (New York: St. Martin's Press, 1990), 66.

Chapter 8   Sex and the Married Man

1. Oswald Schwarz, *The Psychology of Sex* (Hammondsworth, Middlesex, England: Pelican, 1949), 114.

2. Ibid., 139.

3. Paul Tournier, *To Understand Each Other* (Atlanta: John Knox Press, 1987), 46.

4. Ibid.

Chapter 9   Men, Sex, and the Workplace

1. Samuel S. Janus and Cynthia L. Janus, *The Janus Report on Sexual Behavior* (New York: Wiley and Sons, 1993), 365.

2. Michael White, *Los Angeles Times*, 20 May 1993, A7.

3. Louise F. Fitzgerald, "Sexual Harassment: Violence Against Women in the Workplace," *American Psychologist*, October 1993, 1,071.

4. Fitzgerald, "Sexual Harassment," 1,071.

5. *Cosmopolitan*, quoted in "Man and Myth," *Pasadena Star News*, 12 September 1993, D1.

Chapter 10   Religion and Sex

1. Clifford Penner and Joyce Penner, *The Gift of Sex* (Dallas: Word, 1981), 41.

2. Samuel S. Janus and Cynthia L. Janus, *The Janus Report on Sexual Behavior* (New York: Wiley and Sons, 1993), 239.

3. Ibid., 227.

4. Ned Zeman, "The Whoopee Monster," *Newsweek*, 8 March 1993, 51.

5. Janus and Janus, *The Janus Report*, 260.

6. Ibid., 238.

7. Ibid.

8. Ibid., 243.

9. Archibald D. Hart, *Children and Divorce* (Dallas: Word, 1982, 1989).

10. Lewis B. Smedes, *Sex for Christians* (Grand Rapids, Mich.: William B. Eerdmans, 1976), 15.

11. Kenneth Woodward and Patricia King, "When a Pastor Turns Seducer," *Newsweek*, 28 August 1989, 48.

Chapter 11   Creating a Healthy Sexuality

1. Ernest Becker, *The Denial of Death* (New York: The Free Press, 1973), 164.

2. Ibid.

3. Oswald Schwarz, *The Psychology of Sex* (Hammondsworth, Middlesex, England: Penguin Books, 1949), 189.

4. Ibid., 173.

5. Lewis B. Smedes, *Sex for Christians* (Grand Rapids, Mich.: William B. Eerdmans, 1976), 80.

DR. ARCHIBALD HART is the dean of the Graduate School of Psychology at Fuller Theological Seminary in Pasadena, California. Originally from South Africa, Dr. Hart is the author of eighteen books, including *Stress and Your Child, Overcoming Anxiety,* and *The Hidden Link Between Adrenaline and Stress.* He is a highly respected psychologist, widely acclaimed as a lecturer, who has traveled internationally as well as throughout the United States. He and his wife, Kathleen, have three grown daughters and six grandchildren. They reside in Arcadia, California.